Handbook of poisoning in dogs and cats

ALEXANDER CAMPBELL and MICHAEL CHAPMAN

Blackwell
Science

© 2000 A Campbell and M Chapman
Blackwell Science Ltd
Editorial Offices:
Osney Mead, Oxford OX2 0EL
25 John Street, London WC1N 2BL
23 Ainslie Place, Edinburgh EH3 6AJ
350 Main Street, Malden
 MA 02148 5018, USA
54 University Street, Carlton
 Victoria 3053, Australia
10, rue Casimir Delavigne
 75006 Paris, France

Other Editorial Offices:

Blackwell Wissenschafts-Verlag GmbH
Kurfürstendamm 57
10707 Berlin, Germany

Blackwell Science KK
MG Kodenmacho Building
7-10 Kodenmacho Nihombashi
Chuo-ku, Tokyo 104, Japan

The right of the Authors to be identified as
the Authors of this Work has been asserted
in accordance with the Copyright, Designs
and Patents Act 1988.

First published 2000

Typeset and produced by Gray Publishing,
Tunbridge Wells, Kent

The Blackwell Science logo is a
trade mark of Blackwell Science Ltd,
registered at the United Kingdom
Trade Marks Registry

DISTRIBUTORS

 Marston Book Services Ltd
 PO Box 269
 Abingdon
 Oxon OX14 4YN
 (Orders: Tel: 01235 465500
      Fax: 01235 465555)
USA
 Blackwell Science, Inc.
 Commerce Place
 350 Main Street
 Malden, MA 02148 5018
 (Orders: Tel: 800 759 6102
      781 388 8250
    Fax: 781 388 8255)
Canada
 Login Brothers Book Company
 324 Saulteaux Crescent
 Winnipeg, Manitoba R3J 3T2
 (Orders: Tel: 204 837-2987
    Fax: 204 837-3116)
Australia
 Blackwell Science Pty Ltd
 54 University Street
 Carlton, Victoria 3053
 (Orders: Tel: 03 9347 0300
    Fax: 03 9347 5001)

A catalogue record for this title is available
from the British Library
ISBN 0-632-05029-2

For further information on
Blackwell Science, visit our website:
www.blackwell-science.com

Contents

Acknowledgements

This book was planned and written over a considerable period of time and there have been many people involved in its preparation. As editors we would like to thank all those who have made a valuable contribution to the work.

First, we would like to thank Nicky Bates, Jennifer Butler and Mark Colbridge, all members of the National Poisons Information Service (NPIS) in London, for their help in writing some of the monographs in this handbook. Nicky Bates deserves special thanks for her large contribution and for lending her wisdom and experience in matters of book production, indexing and editing. We would also like to thank all the other present and past poisons information specialists of the NPIS in London for their help in 'testing' the book and its contents while cheerfully handling the ever-increasing numbers of veterinary enquiries received over the last 8 years. Their useful comments, suggestions and constructive criticism have been invaluable.

The staff at the sister Veterinary Poisons Information Service in Leeds has been very supportive and we acknowledge in particular the help of Marianne Dawson, Lynne Hodgson, Jane Marsh and Alan Judd.

Thanks are also due to Helaina Checketts, the librarian of the Medical Toxicology Unit, for her help in tracking down and obtaining many of the references used in the preparation of the book.

Nick Edwards, the manager of the NPIS in London and Glyn Volans, the director of the Medical Toxicology Unit, also earn our gratitude for their support and encouragement during the preparation of the book, as do all the members of the VPIS's Veterinary Poisons Information Advisory Group. In particular, we would like to acknowledge the efforts of Dr Tom Gibson, one of the founders of this committee, for his sterling efforts in keeping the issue of poisons information provision for the veterinary profession alive until the issue was resolved. Without him, the VPIS, and certainly this handbook, would probably still not exist.

Finally, we would like to thank both Richard Miles and Antonia Seymour of Blackwell Science for ensuring that our text was finally produced as this book.

AC
MC

Introduction

About this book

This book is intended as a handbook to help veterinary clinicians and their staff to manage cases of poisoning in dogs and cats that are presented to their practices, and perhaps to help answer enquiries about potential poisonings received from concerned pet owners. In writing the book, approximately 15 000 past enquiries received by the Veterinary Poisons Information Service in London (VPISLn) have been reviewed in an attempt to provide information on the agents that are commonly implicated in poisoning or potential poisoning cases in small animals. In addition, there are a small number of entries for agents where poisoning cases are less frequent but where the agent may be very toxic, the clinical effects of rapid onset or unusual, or where the recommended treatment regimen is complicated.

Each agent – or group of agents such as 'anticoagulant rodenticides' – has a separate chapter covering its effects in either the cat or the dog. A few chapters combine the information for both species where the clinical effects and management are identical. Each chapter is designed to provide all the information that should be necessary for the immediate management of a particular case without the need to refer elsewhere for additional information. Hence, for example, the information regarding emetics and absorbents is repeated in each chapter. Thus, cross-referencing has deliberately been kept to a minimum.

Each chapter follows a similar format to enable the user to locate the information required quickly once they are familiar with the layout. This structure is that used for all the major entries in the VPIS 'in-house' database. It has gradually evolved though our experience of handling poisons information enquiries from both the veterinary and medical professions for over three decades.

The work of the VPIS

In April 1992 a veterinary poisons information service was officially launched by the London and Leeds centres of the UK National Poisons Information Service (NPIS). Like all the centres of the NPIS, prior to this date these centres always answered the few enquiries received from the veterinary profession to the best of their ability. However, from the mid- to late-1980s, an increasing demand for veterinary information from these two centres indicated a need for a poisons information service providing animal-specific advice for the veterinary profession.

Discussions between the London and Leeds centres of the NPIS, the British Veterinary Association, the National Office for Animal Health, the British Agrochemicals Association, other animal welfare organisations and representatives of the veterinary pharmaceutical industry opened to debate the issue of animal toxicology and the provision of poisons information. Several studies were initiated and carried out. These concluded that most veterinarians who had used the existing NPIS facilities had found the information provided helpful in managing poisoning cases. It was also considered that expansion of the NPIS remit to cover veterinary toxicology was perhaps the most cost-effective method of starting a veterinary poisons service, since the infrastructure was already in place and the centres had long experience of providing such a service to the medical profession. However, as the NPIS is largely funded by the Department of Health to serve health service professionals only, it was clear that if the service was to continue providing information to the profession, then separate funding would need to be found.

In the spring of 1992 it was decided that the VPIS would be set up to operate from the Leeds and London NPIS centres. The service was advertised as a subscription service to which veterinary practices would need to register on an annual basis and has continued operating in this way. On payment of a small annual fee each practice is offered unlimited access to either centre 24 hours a day. The fee is dependent on the number of veterinary surgeons working in the practice. The service is not public access and is offered only to veterinary surgeons, animal welfare organisations, industry and those involved in veterinary research.

At the start of each enquiry a subscriber number is requested to identify the caller and then the enquiry will be handled. The enquiries are answered by trained information specialists and pharmacists with ready access to a wide variety of sources. These include veterinary toxicology textbooks, past case reports from the literature, and the results and findings of animal laboratory work performed during drug or product testing. There are also human toxicology databases that contain some animal data and there is a database of past cases reported to the VPIS. Additionally, as part of the NPIS, the VPIS has access to a large library of data sheets provided by manufacturers throughout the UK. These are held in commercial confidence but they do provide information about the composition, packaging, physicochemical characteristics and, in some cases, toxicological characteristics of a wide variety of commercially available products or preparations. Access to these data therefore allows the VPIS staff to make some assessment of the potential risks to animals where exposures occur.

The VPIS also has a number of experts to whom referrals can be made when the need arises, and the laboratory facilities of the NPIS are also made available to the VPIS subscribers. Referral to the laboratory is made through the information service staff.

Each enquiry made to the VPIS is recorded at the time of enquiry on a specially designed individual report form. The information collected from the caller would normally cover:

- the source of the enquiry
- the animal concerned (breed, sex, age and also if lactating or pregnant)
- the agent (name, manufacturer, package details, composition)
- the incident (route of exposure, circumstances of exposure, time since exposure)
- the clinical effects (those already present and their timecourse)
- any treatments already instituted
- results and findings of any laboratory or other investigations performed
- the owner's details (name, address) or any case reference.

This 'snapshot' of a case at this particular point of time is vital in allowing some risk assessment to be made before information is provided from the sources mentioned above.

For the majority of the enquiries received the callers are then asked to provide written follow-up information about the cases. Case questionnaires are dispatched within 14 days of the initial information request, together with a reply-paid envelope. These forms request further information about the incident and allow verification of the information recorded at the time of the original enquiry. They also allow outcome of the case to be documented and provide valuable information about how the incident was handled after the VPIS consultation. It is these data that are used to build the 'in-house' database of past case reports that has proved so valuable in answering enquiries. A facsimile of this form is to be found in Appendix 2 of this book.

When a large number of reports about a specific agent in a specific animal are collected, the information is used, together with what is available in the literature, to compile the type of monograph found in this book. These represent a distillation of the data that are currently available on the agent in question, but more importantly they are based largely on past case experience. The sections for each entry allow information on the relevant aspect of the case, whether clinical effects, potential fatal dose, management or kinetics, to be accessed and delivered rapidly. The callers will therefore usually be provided with information within minutes of telephone contact.

Loosely categorised, the sections cover the following.

The agent(s)

This section covers description and classification of the agent where appropriate. For animals and plants the common location may be described. For drugs, household products and pesticides, there will be information about the usual presentation and composition of the products, including strengths available. There may be information about the intended use and, in the case of drugs that have a veterinary application, the recommended dosage.

Incidence of poisoning

This section outlines the number of enquiries that may be received by the VPIS about the agent per annum. This is to provide some idea of likely occurrence. There may also be some outline information about the number of cases with a fatal outcome or those that remain asymptomatic.

Recommended dosage

This provides the recommended dosage regimen for drugs that have veterinary application in the species under discussion.

Toxicity

These sections outline what is known about the toxicity of the agent. They will usually include some LD_{50} or lowest fatal dose data from the literature, together with similar information from past VPIS cases. There may be also some case reports from the VPIS database or the literature. These will be included where they provide detailed illustration of a serious case.

Mechanism of toxicity

Where included, this section will outline the mechanism of toxicity in the species in question.

Kinetics and metabolism

This section is included to provide data on the absorption, metabolism and elimination of the agent. This may be useful in determining how long the animal may need to be observed or treated, and also in determining whether certain management protocols should be instituted.

Clinical effects

This section describes the likely clinical effects resulting from exposure. They will generally be categorised into those that are likely to occur frequently and those that might occur more rarely or in more severe poisonings. In some cases, there may be some information on common post-mortem findings.

Treatment

These sections outline a suggested management protocol. There will usually be some guidelines as to what would constitute an exposure that necessitates some form of treatment. Dose regimens for emetics and adsorbents will be detailed where appropriate. Where other drugs or antidotes are used in treatment, the indications and dosage regimens will be provided. There may be some suggestion for minimum observation times.

Where laboratory analyses may be useful in determining treatment, these will be provided.

References

These sections provide details of the literature papers and articles that have been used in the compilation of the monograph and provide a useful reading list for those wishing to pursue further study or investigation into a particular topic.

Review of work to date

Since the launch of the VPIS in 1992, the two branches of the service have kept a record of every enquiry they have received. When collated these give an indication of the types of poisonings that are relatively common-place and those that are more rare but that are potentially serious when they do occur. Sadly, no national statistics on the occurrence of poisoning cases in animals are collected and the full extent of the problem is therefore unknown. These VPIS data probably do not reflect the national occurrence for the following reasons. First, not all practices in the UK use the VPIS. Second, those that do probably do not contact the service about all the poisoning or suspected poisoning cases that present to their premises. Many will only call about more complex cases, those where there are unexpected or serious clinical effects or those where data are lacking from other sources. However, when compared with one another, the experience of each centre is very similar.

In 1992 the VPIS London centre received a total of 951 enquiries. By 1998 the total enquiries handled per annum had reached 4292. A total of 68% of these enquiries involve exposures or potential exposures in dogs and 17% in cats. The remaining enquiries concern exposures in horses, livestock, miscellaneous and other species.

The most common enquiries received during this time are listed in order below.

- Ibuprofen ingestion by dogs
- Difenacoum ingestion by dogs
- Bromadiolone ingestion by dogs
- Paracetamol ingestion by dogs
- Metaldehyde ingestion by dogs
- Unknown agent exposures in dogs
- Oral contraceptives ingestion by dogs
- Salbutamol exposures in dogs
- Borax ingestion by dogs
- Adder bites to dogs

- Permethrin exposures in cats
- Chocolate ingestion by dogs
- Glyphosate exposures in dogs
- Diclofenac sodium ingestion by dogs
- Bone meal ingestion by dogs
- Paraquat exposures in dogs
- Coumatetralyl ingestion by dogs
- Unknown agent exposures in cats
- Fertiliser ingestion by dogs
- Alphachloralose ingestion by dogs.

As can be seen, many of these common enquires concern pesticides including anticoagulant rodenticides (e.g. difenacoum, bromadiolone, coumatetralyl), molluscicides (metaldehyde), and insecticides (permethrin). Drugs commonly encountered in the home environment including the analgesics or anti-inflammatory drugs ibuprofen, diclofenac sodium and paracetamol are the other common type of enquiry.

The broad group 'medicines' comprises the largest category of enquiries each year, accounting for approximately 30% of calls. Agrochemicals are the next most numerous category representing 26% of the total calls. Of these anticoagulant rodenticides comprise the largest sub-category at 11% of the total calls. Other calls relate to industrial chemicals (12%), household products (11%), plants and fungi (13%), and the remainder concern animal bites or stings, micro-organism ingestion (blue–green algae) and general enquiries.

Between 3% and 6% of the VPISLn enquiries concern cases later reported to have fatal outcomes. The agents most commonly implicated in these fatal cases are:

- Metaldehyde in dogs
- Paraquat in dogs and cats
- Anticoagulant rodenticides in dogs (e.g. difenacoum, brodifacoum and bromadiolone)
- Blue–green algae in dogs
- Paracetamol in cats.

All these agents are covered by monographs in this handbook.

The increasing usage of the VPIS centres by veterinary surgeons in the UK demonstrates that the service continues to provide a valuable and reliable source of information on animal toxicology. With increased usage it is possible for more case data to be routinely collected and therefore for the quality of the information provided to be updated and improved constantly.

The continued surveillance of all enquiries undertaken by both centres places the VPIS in a unique position to alert the veterinary profession, industry, regulatory authorities and other interested parties about agents that are causing concern. It also allows trends in animal poisoning and its management to be monitored.

Gastric decontamination

Introduction

The removal of any unabsorbed poison from the patient is an obvious and logical step. Specific entries in this book deal with the cases, perhaps exceptional, where it is necessary to decontaminate the exterior of the body (e.g. the skin, eyes). The gut lumen is obviously both more problematic to remove a poison from and yet likely to require at least the consideration of emptying in the majority of cases.

Techniques have been developed for removing material from all the various portions of the alimentary tract, but it is the possibility of emptying the stomach of as yet unabsorbed material that is of the greatest potential benefit and that also requires prompt action on the clinician's part. (For a discussion of techniques for other portions of the gastrointestinal tract, see Chapman and Campbell, 2001.) While emptying the stomach of any burden of unabsorbed poison may be obvious and logical, it has been the subject of recent intense debate in human medicine. Snodgrass (1996, p. 971) states: 'Published clinical trials of [human] patients with oral overdose ingestions do *not* show that induced emesis (usually with ipecac syrup; much less frequently used is apomorphine or a mild liquid detergent) improves patient outcome compared with the use of oral or gastrically instilled activated charcoal' [emphasis in original]. However in the cat and the dog, if not in all veterinary species, the dangers from aspiration do not in practice appear to be as great as those in man. Indeed, spontaneous vomition in the dog is so frequent that it should probably not be considered as 'pathological' in the majority of cases. Also, consideration (in the absence of formal trials specific to veterinary species) has to be given to the relative ease with which vomiting can be induced in the dog and the cat, compared with the greater difficulty of inducing ingestion of activated charcoal mixtures.

Gastric emptying

Two methods are available, the choice likely to be forced to a large extent by the patient's clinical condition.

Both methods obviously aim to prevent or reduce further exposure to the toxicant by removing it from the body. The success of the method will depend on the delay between ingestion and gastric emptying and on the nature of the poison.

There is no agreement amongst authors as to when gastric emptying becomes futile, and indeed there are no simple studies upon which to base advice. After 4 hours though, the greater part of stomach contents will have moved on into the duodenum and, if not yet absorbed from the gastrointestinal tract, will be beyond the reach of gastric emptying. Obviously, this may not apply to larger material. However, the mechanical objects described in this text (thermometers, batteries) are not ones that would indicate gastrotomy for their removal, nor is the accumulation of large amounts of poorly chewed plant material usually a problem in the cat or dog.

There is general agreement that up to 2 hours after ingestion a significant amount of material is likely to be still present in the stomach and to justify attempts at its removal. Between 2 and 4 hours, a clinical judgement has to be made upon the basis of the suspected toxicant, its physical form and the amount likely to have been ingested.

As a very general rule of thumb, the induction of emesis should be considered until at least 3 hours after ingestion. On the other hand, the risks of gastric lavage mean that (unless the patient is in any event unconscious) careful consideration should be given as to whether its benefits are likely to outweigh the risks after 2 hours. However, for each poison discussed in this book more specific guidelines relating to elapsed time and advisability of gastric emptying are given (see specific monograph chapters).

The physical form of the poison (large tablets as against a solution, for example) will affect the time ingested material is available in the stomach to be recovered. The chemical nature of the toxicant contained in the poison may also have its affect. Local anaesthetics (e.g. cocaine) tend to pass from the stomach slowly, while other compounds (e.g. alcohol) can be absorbed directly from the stomach.

Emesis

Emesis is contra-indicated:

- If the patient is unconscious, is very depressed or has a poor swallow reflex. Consideration should be given to the time that may elapse before the emetic takes effect and the apparent speed of deterioration of the patient's consciousness, if the latter is obvious.
- If the patient is susceptible to seizures.
- If the poison was corrosive or caustic. Not only may the poison cause more damage as it retransits the oropharynx and oesophagus, but the act of vomition may rupture these already weakened tissues.
- If the poison is of low viscosity, or in a low-viscosity vehicle; e.g. petroleum distillates.

The following points may influence the choice of emetic, or how emesis is induced:

- Apomorphine can have an additive effect in opiate poisonings. However, reversing agents specific to this opiate effect are readily available. A suitable reversing agent should be held for use if necessary following apomorphine, e.g. naloxone.
- Xylazine is also sedative. Again, a specific reversing agent is available should this prove to be a problem, i.e. atipamezole. A suitable reversing agent should be held for use if necessary following xylazine.

The using of 'a crystal' of washing soda (see for example Humphreys, 1988, p. 13) seems to be almost apocryphal both in veterinary texts and among the practising veterinary profession. The author, and many of his colleagues were all well aware of the method but reported no experience of it, preferring to use the surer administration of an injectable emetic. The method has been retained in this text as there seems no clear evidence of its lack of efficacy; washing soda is still relatively commonly available; and, of all the 'household remedies' (detergent, mustard, etc.) it is at least one that does not have major questions about its safety. Washing soda may also be kept more readily available in visit bags, etc. than controlled substances such as apomorphine. The major hazard with lay administration is that the wrong compound might be administered: washing soda is sodium carbonate (caustic soda – sodium hydroxide – must obviously not be administered, and baking soda – sodium bicarbonate – will have little effect).

Syrup of Ipecacuanha (ipecac syrup) is generally considered without the major hazards associated with the 'household' emetics discussed above. However, it is rarely available outside a practice setting, and has few if any advantages over the injectable agents. Indeed there are two possible adverse effects associated with its use that should be considered. First, it can cause CNS depression (especially if the dose has to be repeated). Second, it can cause diarrhoea, risking dehydration of the patient if untreated. Additionally, there is often an appreciable delay before the emetic actions are observed.

Gastric lavage

Gastric lavage is contra-indicated:

- If emesis can be safely carried out and there is no indication for administering activated charcoal. (The effects of emetics will delay the opportunity for administering an absorbent, whereas activated charcoal can be given by stomach tube immediately after (or even during) gastric lavage.)

The following points may influence the choice of gastric lavage, or how it is carried out:

- There is a significantly increased risk of perforating the alimentary tract following the ingestion of caustic or corrosive poisons.
- In smaller or younger animals with vigorous use of lavage, consideration should be given to maintenance of body temperature.

Gastric lavage should be performed in the unconscious patient. Thus, general anaesthesia may be required.

Water, saline, or a charcoal slurry may be used. The latter prevents good visualisation of what is being removed from the stomach, but has the advantage that if any stomach content is forced on beyond the stomach (into the duodenum) it will be combined with activated charcoal.

The steps are as follows:

1. A cuffed endo-tracheal tube should first be inserted and the cuff inflated.
2. While, theoretically, a double bore tube might be used for gastric lavage, these are not commonly available, not least in the range of sizes necessary. Instead the widest bore single tube available should be used. This should have side openings to reduce the risk of blockage.
3. The animal should be measured from the tip of the nose to the xiphisternum and this length marked clearly on the tube. The tube should then be introduced up to that mark.
4. Lavage fluid should then be introduced down the tube. This must be done gently as excessive pressure will force poison into the duodenum. The simplest way of controlling pressure is to attach a funnel to the end of the tube and fill this so that fluid enters under the effects of gravity alone. As a rough guide 10 ml/kg body weight of fluid should be measured out for each wash, and as much of this used as is clinically appropriate.
    Tilting the animal (nose downwards) or lowering the head relative to the body (partially over the side of the table) once the tube is in, but before lavage, will further reduce contamination of the oropharynx and thus the entry to the trachea.
5. Lowering the exterior end of the tube will then cause emptying by gravity. Suction can be used if required and available.
6. The process should be repeated several times; on the final washes the fluid coming out should be clear and free of any particulate matter.
7. Consideration should be given to then using the same tube to place a slurry of activated charcoal in the stomach (see next section).
8. Care should be taken on withdrawing the tube, and the rear of the mouth cleaned manually if necessary, before removal of the endo-tracheal tube.

Absorption

Activated charcoal will absorb many (though not all) poisons. Specific advice is given in the relevant chapters of this book; for example, that activated charcoal is considered of little benefit in metaldehyde poisoning.

Animals may be 'drenched' with a slurry of charcoal if conscious, though this is neither easy, nor usually accomplished without much of the slurry being shaken over attendant and the surrounding area. In paediatrics, mixtures of charcoal and ice cream have been used, and proprietary preparations of claimed improved palatability are available, but there is apparently no published method demonstrating improved charcoal palatability in animals.

A slurry should be made by mixing 10–20 g of activated charcoal in 100 ml of tap water.

Following gastric lavage, charcoal may easily be administered by stomach tube. It may be administered following emetics provided 'anti-emetic cover' is given to counteract the effect of the emetic.

The use of activated charcoal is contra-indicated if it is desired to give medication immediately by the oral route – the charcoal will absorb most medicines, rendering them ineffective. Where this is a factor in specific treatment protocols, this is dealt with in individual chapters.

Repeat doses of activated charcoal are advised if the suspected toxic agent is likely to cause gastric stasis, is one that will undergo enterohepatic recirculation, or has a low volume of distribution.

Activated charcoal is manufactured by the destructive distillation of (vegetable) organic matter. Ten kilogrammes of activated charcoal have surface area of around 1 km^2. It is essential that chemically activated charcoal is used to ensure that the product has the maximum ability to absorb toxicants.

General considerations

As soon as the patient is under treatment, and especially after gastric decontamination has been carried out, it is essential to ensure that further ingestion of the (suspected) poison is prevented. Vomit should be cleared away to prevent re-eating or eating by another animal. Access to the original source of poison should be stopped (for the patient and for other potential patients!). It may be necessary to prevent self-grooming (or grooming by other animals). Prevention of self-grooming is perhaps most easily achieved by use of an 'Elizabethan collar'.

Consideration should be given to the retention of samples of vomit and/or stomach contents as these are produced by the animal (see chapter on 'Laboratory Sampling and Analysis').

References

Chapman MJ and Campbell A (2001). *Veterinary Toxicology*. Oxford: Blackwell Science (in press).

Humphreys DJ (1988). *Veterinary Toxicology* (third edition). London: Baillière Tindall, pp. 13–14.

Snodgrass WR (1996). Clinical Toxicology. In CJ Klaassen (ed.), *Casarett and Doull's Toxicology – The Basic Science of Poisons*. London: McGraw-Hill, pp. 969–986.

Laboratory sampling and analysis and sending samples by post

Introduction

Appropriate laboratory tests are discussed in individual chapters of this book. For a discussion of investigation of cases where the agent is unknown see Chapman and Campbell (2001).

Obtaining suitable specimens for submission is generally no different from taking samples from any other patient. The one major exception is the submission of induced vomitus for analysis. This, however, will generally be produced secondary to the induction of emesis as a prophylactic measure. Methods of inducing emesis are detailed in the chapter on gastric decontamination.

Personal safety must also be kept in mind. Significant amounts of poisons are unlikely to be present in body fluids or tissues, but it is possible. The most likely sources of large amounts of toxicants are in the case of skin contamination of an animal and if the original poison or its packaging have to be handled.

The two major issues to be borne in mind are legalistic ones. First, it is always wise to presume that any suspicion or accusation of poisoning may lead to litigation, and thus sampling and analysis should be capable of withstanding forensic scrutiny. Second, while practitioners do routinely submit samples to laboratories by post, in poisoning cases the nature of the samples and the laboratories used will tend to vary from the routine and thus some reflection on the relevant regulations regarding transmission of pathological specimens is in order.

Sampling

Samples must be taken, stored and transported so that their provenance is not only known but can be proved to be known.

As those involved might be called to give oral evidence before a court, the number of people involved should be minimised. (It is always worth viewing any step in a procedure that may lead to litigation from an adversarial 'gamesmanship' point of view. It is unlikely, and would be considered time-wasting, to call everyone who had handled a sample, merely to say that they had handled it. Indeed, a tribunal might be tempted to penalise a party calling so many witnesses by ordering costs against them. The one situation where this would be worthwhile would be where it became impossible to prove the 'continuity of the evidence'. There was a gap in the record of it being handled. Thus it is never wise to presume that 'such and such' will not happen. It is the more likely to happen if the record is thin!) In many situations there will be no necessity for more than two people to be directly involved. The clinician can take a sample and before leaving the room seal that sample in a packet. This can be sent, in outer packaging, to the laboratory. There the final sealed container can be entered by the laboratory scientist who is to perform the analysis. For this to work smoothly requires several precautions.

- Containers are rarely large enough for proper labelling. They should, however, be uniquely labelled. The sampler's initials and a number are the minimum, with – if space allows – a date. A list can then be drawn up with the sample reference details and a more precise description of the sample.
- The law is slow. Always give full dates (including the year). However memorable the case, do not rely on remembering anything some years later.
- 'Contemporaneous' notes carry great weight. That is what was written at the time, without the benefit of reflection. Thus hand-written observations may be of greater value than a perfectly edited typescript. Record the time notes are taken. It is better that they are a precise time after the event than 'nearly' at the same time.
- Samples may become mislabelled. It is even easier to suggest that they have become so. Never label the part of the container (e.g. the screw-bottle top) that is least associated with the sample (e.g. the bottle contents).
- Warn the laboratory before they receive the sample not only what is in the sample, but that litigation is at least a possibility and draw their attention to the fact that samples are 'sealed'. Unless the laboratory is used to this, it will be best to discuss it by telephone to ensure that the matter is fully understood.
- Seal samples simply, but adequately. A simple paper envelope, closed with matt 'Scotch' tape will be tamper-evident. The tape can then be 'sealed' by signing across it. The addition of a practice rubber stamp and/or date stamp across the tape will facilitate identification and assure as to authenticity. Always presume the outer packaging will be opened by someone other than the intended final recipient!
- If litigation seems likely, in fairness you must work as far as possible to assist both sides. To take an extreme example: if litigation is certain concerning heavy metal poisoning and half a litre of vomitus is available for analysis, of which only a few tens of millilitres will be required, then there is no reason not to submit a 100 ml sample, dividing the remainder into a second (identical) 100 ml sample and the residue (of say 300 ml). The latter two samples can then (after sealing) be frozen. The second 100 ml is there to be 'taken up' by the other party if they wish to have it analysed. The residue can be used if the two independent laboratories come to contradictory results. At the

other extreme, blood samples from a neonatal kitten are likely to be all used for clinical management with probably little scope for retaining any surplus sample.

• Guidelines such as this are general. If litigation is anticipated, consider asking advice from the laboratory you will submit material to, professional associations, any prosecuting authority, the client (if relevant) and your professional defence society/insurer.

Posting

In the UK 'letter post' and 'parcel post' are operated by separate entities. There are also a multitude of organisations offering courier services. Thus, it is no longer possible to cite 'the postal regulations'.

Specific contact should be made with the intended carrier as to whether, and if so under what conditions, they are willing to carry samples. Couriers normally display contact numbers prominently on their packages. It should not be forgotten that similar considerations apply to 'informal' courier methods (bikes, taxis, etc.).

A member of the public must not send any pathological specimen except under the instructions of a veterinary surgeon or recognised laboratory, in which case appropriate packaging and instructions must be provided.

Consideration of the following points will usually lead to only one likely solution:

• *Are the samples themselves a toxic hazard?* It will rarely be the case that concentration and/or sample size will mean that there is any significant amount of suspected poison in a sample. If, however, the suspected poison itself is to be submitted, then different considerations may apply. If, for whatever reason, it is considered that there is a significant toxic hazard, then specific advice on packaging must be sought.

• *Are samples likely to carry infection?* While the answer to this is probably 'no' (and could even be made 'no', by, for example, fixing tissues), it is generally best to presume that the answer is 'yes' and treat all material as carrying some risk. Though not mandatory, in the post-HIV era, it is now reassuring to carriers to actually clearly mark samples as of *veterinary* origin!

• *Is any likely infection in WHO group 4?* If it is, then material must *not* be sent by post or similar methods. (Group 4 agents are of marked pathogenicity and will rarely be associated with suspected small animal poisonings.)

International regulations on the transport (both domestic and international) of pathological specimens (including group 1 to group 3 pathogen material) by air are being applied to UK carriage by the Civil Aviation Authority (CAA) and the International Air Transport Association (IATA). (All major airlines are IATA members.)

As virtually any domestic package could be transported by air (if only by accidental misdirection), and a surprising number actually are, then these regulations form a useful if stringent minimum. That minimum is compliance with U.N. 602 packaging requirements. The Royal Mail will supply a list of approved U.N. 602 packaging suppliers on request. The basis of the requirement is that:

'The system consists of three layers as follows:

Primary receptacle

A labelled primary watertight, leak-proof receptacle containing the sample. The receptacle is wrapped in enough absorbent material to absorb all fluid in the case of breakage.

Secondary receptacle

A second durable, watertight, leak-proof receptacle to close and protect the primary receptacle(s). Several wrapped primary receptacles may be placed in one secondary receptacle. Sufficient additional absorbent material must be used to cushion multiple primary receptacles.

Outer shipping package

The secondary package is placed in an outer shipping package, which protects it from outside influences, such as physical damage and water while in transit. Information concerning the sample, such as data forms, letters and other types of information that identify or describe the sample, should be taped to the outside of the secondary receptacle.'

The regulations are being introduced in the UK at the time that this book goes to press. However, it *seems* likely that:

- purpose-made clinical sample containers should in general comply as 'primary receptacles'
- 'enough absorbent material' should be self-explanatory
- a sealable plastic bag is likely to satisfy the requirement for the 'secondary receptacle'
- sufficient wadding/packing must then be used in the outer container
- a tough cardboard box should satisfy the requirement for the 'outer shipping package'.

Previous guidance, which remains valid, is that:

- individual containers should not exceed 50 ml
- the outer packaging must be clearly labelled
  - o '[VETERINARY] PATHOLOGICAL SPECIMEN – FRAGILE WITH CARE'
  - o with the sender's address
  - o with contact telephone numbers for sender and addressee
- all regulations change – always check with your local carrier.

Conclusion

In the words of Lorgue *et al.* (1996, at p.25):

Laboratories can only operate effectively if they receive high quality samples, in good conditions and of sufficient quantity, accompanied by complete and accurate documentation.

References

Chapman, MJ and Campbell A (2001). *Veterinary Toxicology.* Oxford: Blackwell Science (in press).

Lorgue G, Lechenet J and Rivière A (1996). MJ Chapman (ed.), *Clinical Veterinary Toxicology.* Oxford: Blackwell Science, pp. 25 (translated from French).

Benzalkonium chloride

Type of product

Benzalkonium chloride (BAC, alkyldimethylbenzylammonium chloride) is a quaternary ammonium compound (QAC), which is classified as a cationic detergent. Cationic detergents dissociate in aqueous solution to produce an active complex ion and a small inactive one. They are used mainly as disinfectants and rarely as simple cleaning agents.

Presentation

In past VPIS cases the benzalkonium chloride-containing product to which cats are most commonly exposed is Dettox® (Reckitt & Colman), which contains 2–3.5%. Less commonly, Zoflora® (Thornton & Ross) is the agent involved. This contains benzalkonium chloride at a concentration of 3.8%.

Occurrence of poisoning incidences

Since 1992 the VPIS has received over 20 enquiries per year concerning accidental exposure of cats to disinfectant or multi-surface cleaner products containing benzalkonium chloride. These cases usually occur when the animals accidentally walk across treated surfaces or fall in buckets of the cleaners. There are cases where cats have drunk quantities of the undiluted solutions.

They often develop the signs of buccal irritation as a result of grooming themselves after dermal exposures.

Toxicity

The primary effects of benzalkonium chloride are due to its irritancy. Systemic effects are uncommon.

According to the literature:

- Dermal absorption is minimal but may occur through prolonged contact on broken skin. Chemical burns have been reported following the use of an undiluted 17% solution of benzalkonium chloride as an electrical conductant during normal ECG monitoring in cats and dogs (Bilbrey et al., 1989).

In the experience of VPISLn:

- No fatal cases have been reported.
- One 2-year-old 2 kg domestic short-haired cat consumed 2 ml of a disinfectant. Within 12 hours the animal had salivation, anorexia,

pyrexia, abdominal tenderness and severe oral ulceration. The cat was managed supportively with intravenous fluids, corticosteroids and antibiotics and made a rapid recovery. The ulcers took 7 days to heal (VPISLn case 94/31849).

- A 4-month-old domestic short-haired cat fell into a bucket of disinfectant. The animal evidently consumed some of the fluid and also inhaled some. It became drowsy, anorexic and pyrexic. It had severe lung congestion, severe ulceration of the mouth and tongue and the skin was red and inflamed. After washing it was given steroids, antibiotics, frusemide and intravenous fluid support and made a full recovery (VPISLn case 94/125099).

Clinical effects

Onset of effects is usually within 12 hours, but will be more rapid following exposure to more concentrated solutions.

Ingestion or oral exposure following grooming after dermal exposure may cause salivation, vomiting, inappetence, diarrhoea and ulceration of the tongue and oral mucosa (which may be severe). Dehydration and anorexia may occur. In more severe cases there may be depression, pyrexia and respiratory effects including dyspnoea, hyperpnoea and coughing.

On the skin, particularly of the feet, there may be erythema, inflammation, ulceration, hair loss and contact dermatitis. Concentrated solutions may cause chemical burns.

Benzalkonium chloride is also irritant to the eyes and can produce severe injury.

Treatment

Emesis is best avoided because these products are usually foamy and there is a risk of foam aspiration if vomiting occurs. Adsorbents may be given if the exposure was recent. However, endoscopic evaluation of injury to the gastrointestinal tract may be required and in these cases adsorbents should not be given.

Adsorbents:

(a) Activated charcoal   Dose: 2 g/kg body weight orally
(b) BCK granules®   Dose: 6–18 g orally.

The animal should be thoroughly washed and then collared to limit self-grooming and further ingestion of benzalkonium chloride. The eyes should also be irrigated. They may be stained with fluorescein and examined for corneal injury if appropriate.

Treatment thereafter is symptomatic and supportive. Rehydration may be required and a bland diet is recommended. Antibiotics and steroids may also be given. Atropine may be administered if there is severe salivation. The animal should be monitored for development of respiratory effects.

References and further reading

VPIS (London) past cases up to 98/13298.

Bilbrey SA, Dulisch ML and Stallings B (1989). Chemical burns caused by benzalkonium chloride in eight surgical patients. *Journal of the American Animal Hospital Association* **25**, 31–34.

Coppock RW, Mostom MS and Lille LE (1988). The toxicology of detergents, bleaches, antiseptics and disinfectants in small animals. *Veterinary and Human Toxicology* **30(5)**, 463–473.

Kore AM and Kiesche-Nesselrodt A (1990). Toxicology of household cleaning products and disinfectants. *Veterinary Clinics of North America: Small Animal Practice* **20(2)**, 525–537.

Trapani M, Brooks DL and Tillman PC (1982). Quaternary ammonium toxicosis in cats. *Laboratory Animal Science* **32(5)**, 520–522.

Dichlorophen

Type of product

Anthelmintic used for the treatment of *Dipylidium* and *Taenia* infection in cats and dogs.

Presentation

This is usually available in tablet preparations only. Strengths of tablets available are 250 mg, 500 mg, and 750 mg.

Some preparations contain piperazine in combination.

Occurrence of poisoning incidences

Since the launch of the VPIS in 1992 the London centre has received between six and 30 enquiries per year regarding dichlorophen ingestion in cats and dogs. Over 75% of these cases involve cats. All cases reported have exhibited clinical effects, but this may be attributable to the fact that effects had occurred at therapeutic doses and had therefore caused some concern.

Recommended dosage

200 mg/kg body weight for management of *Dipylidium* and *Taenia* infection. Use is contra-indicated in cats less than 6 months of age.

Toxicity

According to the literature:

- No fatal dose has been reported.
- A dose of 69.4 mg/kg body weight produced hyperaesthesia, drooling, ataxia and anorexia in one cat.
- Some animals exhibit signs of toxicity at the therapeutic dose.

In the experience of the VPISLn:

- Effects have been seen at doses as low as 62.5 mg/kg body weight.
- One fatal case attributed to dichlorophen alone. A 16-year-old cat had one 750 mg tablet. Within 12 hours the animal developed ataxia, hyperaesthesia and excessive salivation. The animal was treated supportively with fluids and atropine and after apparent recovery, relapsed and was euthanased (VPISLn case 94/125078).
- Poisoning has also arisen from dosing of 500 mg/week for 2 weeks (VPISLn case 92/95921).

Clinical effects

Onset of effects is usually within 3 hours but sometimes up to 12 hours. Duration of effects may be 2–3 days.

Common effects are vomiting, salivation, ataxia, incoordination, anorexia, tachycardia, lethargy, pyrexia, hyperaesthesia and in severe cases collapse. Other less commonly observed effects include inappetence, hyperventilation, dilated pupils, borborygmi, dyspnoea and disorientation.

Treatment

Gastric decontamination should be considered for any excess of the therapeutic dose (200 mg/kg). Although a small number of animals become unwell with doses below this, there is no method of identifying susceptible individuals.

If within 2 hours of ingestion, induce vomiting or perform gastric lavage, and then administer adsorbents.

Emetics:

(a) Xylazine	Dose:	0.2 mg/kg body weight i.v.; 0.5–1 mg/kg body weight i.m.
(b) Ipecacuanha	Dose:	1–3 ml/kg body weight orally
(c) Soda crystal.		

Adsorbents:

(a) Activated charcoal	Dose:	1–3 g/kg body weight orally
(b) BCK granules®	Dose:	6–18 g orally.

Treatment is essentially symptomatic and supportive as there is no specific antidote. It is essential to monitor the body temperature and institute cooling measures if necessary.

Atropine may be given for hypersalivation, but is best avoided in pyrexic animals.

References and further reading

VPIS (London) past cases up to 97/107258.

Edwards HG (1987). Adverse reactions to dichlorophen in cats. *Veterinary Record* **121(6)**, 136.

Goodwin JL (1987). Adverse reactions to dichlorophen in cats. *Veterinary Record* **121(7)**, 23–24.

Ethylene glycol

Type of product

Ethylene glycol is most commonly encountered in antifreeze, screenwash or, more rarely, de-icers. Most antifreezes available contain ethylene glycol or methanol.

Presentation

Antifreeze is available as a liquid to be added to water in engine radiators to prevent freezing and improve hot weather performance, the usual final dilution being 1:3 or 1:4.

Occurrence of poisoning incidence

Since 1992 the VPIS has received a small number of enquiries regarding ingestion of ethylene glycol by companion animals. Approximately 10% of these cases involved cats. In these feline cases, all presented with severe clinical effects and outcomes were fatal in all but 8% of cases.

Ethylene glycol poisoning is more commonly reported in the winter months.

Toxicity

According to the literature:

- The lethal dose of ethylene glycol in cats is 1.5 ml/kg body weight.
- In 25 cases of ingestion of ethylene glycol in cats the mortality rate was 96% (Rowland, 1987).

Mechanism of toxicity

The major toxic agent in ethylene glycol poisoning is not the parent compound but the metabolites produced by the action of alcohol dehydrogenase on the parent compound. Alcohol dehydrogenase converts ethylene glycol to glycoaldehyde. This is then metabolised to glycolic acid, which appears to be the principal cause of the acidosis. One of the metabolites of glycolic acid is oxalate, which causes renal damage and hypocalcaemia by binding to calcium to form calcium oxalate, crystals of which appear in the urine. The aldehydes (glycoaldehyde, glycolic acid and glyoxylate) may inhibit oxidative phosphorylation and respiration. Glycolic acid is metabolised to glycine, which is metabolised to hippurate.

Kinetics

Ethylene glycol is rapidly absorbed from the gastrointestinal tract. The half-life of ethylene glycol in cats is shorter than in dogs and the onset of the various clinical effects may be more rapid in cats. This may account for the lower fatal dose and higher mortality in cats compared to dogs.

Clinical effects

Stage 1 (30 minutes–12 hours): central nervous system signs, including vomiting, ataxia, tachycardia, weakness and convulsions. Also polydipsia, polyuria, dehydration, tachypnoea, acidosis and hypothermia.

Stage 2 (12–24 hours): cardiopulmonary signs including tachypnoea, tachycardia, pulmonary oedema, hyperaemia and congestion. There may be transient recovery followed by anorexia, severe depression, coma and convulsions.

Stage 3 (24–72 hours): renal system signs including oliguria, azotaemia and/ or uraemia, vomiting, anorexia and severe depression. Renal failure indicates a poor prognosis.

Recovery may take 3–4 weeks. However, in some cases there may be irreversible renal tubular damage.

The longer the time to treatment, the less favourable the prognosis. Animals that have improving clinical signs after 10–16 hours of treatment have a favourable prognosis. However, in most cases unless the ingestion was witnessed, animals usually present in the third stage of poisoning and in these animals the prognosis is poor.

Laboratory findings

(a) Increased osmolality (normal 280–310 mOsm/kg). An osmolality raised by as much as 60 mOsm/kg is typical of ethylene glycol poisoning.
(b) Increased anion gap (normal 10–12 mEq/L). An anion gap >40–50 mEq/L is typical of ethylene glycol poisoning.
(c) Acidosis, pH usually <7.3. Urine pH usually <6.5.
(d) Renal damage: raised urea and creatinine, low urine specific gravity, calcium oxalate crystals (may appear within 5 hours of ingestion), proteinuria, glucosuria, haematuria and albuminuria. Calcium oxalate crystals are light yellow, arranged in rosettes, sheaves or prisms and are birefringent (transmit light unequally in different directions) in polarised light.
(e) Hyperglycaemia, hypocalcaemia, hyperphosphataemia, hyperkalaemia.
(f) Neutrophil leucocytosis, eosinopaenia (Johnson *et al.*, 1979).
(g) Raised ethylene glycol concentrations in blood and urine.
(h) Hippurate and oxalate detected in urine.

Post-mortem findings

(a) Gastrointestinal tract: gastric mucosa haemorrhagic and hyperaemic.
(b) Pulmonary hyperaemia and oedema.
(c) Kidney: pale, swollen with grey or yellow streaks, particularly near the corticomedullary junction. Oxalate crystals are usually present in the kidney. In animals that survive, regenerating renal tubules are dilated and lined with flattened tubular epithelium.

Diagnosis

Ethylene glycol poisoning may be mistaken for head trauma, encephalitis, acute gastroenteritis, pancreatitis, ketoacidotic diabetes mellitus and acute renal failure from other causes. Diagnosis is based on history, clinical signs and laboratory data. Abdominal palpation may be painful due to renal oedema. Ethylene glycol poisoning should be suspected in any animal with the following:

(a) acute onset of signs
(b) raised urea, creatinine and other nitrogenous compounds in the blood (azotaemia or uraemia)
(c) low or fixed urine specific gravity (Grauer and Thrall, 1982).

Treatment

Therapy for ethylene glycol is principally aimed at blocking the action of alcohol dehydrogenase to prevent the formation of the toxic metabolites. This is achieved by administration of the preferred substrate, ethanol, which allows renal excretion of the unmetabolised parent compound.

4-Methylpyrazole (4-MP, fomepizole), a direct inhibitor of the enzyme alcohol dehydrogenase, has been suggested as an alternative therapy to ethanol on the grounds of a lack of adverse effects and slower elimination. Clinical reports suggest that 4-MP is successful in treating ethylene glycol intoxication in dogs, but it has been shown to be less effective than ethanol in cats poisoned with ethylene glycol and is therefore not recommended.

If within 2 hours of ingestion, induce vomiting or perform gastric lavage. Adsorbents are not useful.

Emetics:

(a) Xylazine   Dose: 0.2 mg/kg body weight i.v.;
     0.5–1 mg/kg body weight i.m.
(b) Ipecacuanha   Dose: 1–3 ml/kg body weight orally
(c) Soda crystal.

Monitor pH and renal function. Correct acidosis with sodium bicarbonate (see below). Fluids should be given to ensure adequate hydration and a good urine output. Central venous pressure and renal output should be monitored in cats with renal dysfunction because of the risk of fluid overload and subsequent pulmonary oedema. Mannitol can be used in a well-hydrated animal to produce an osmotic diuresis and reduce renal oedema.

Dose: 0.25–0.5 g/kg body weight, i.v. over 5–10 minutes.

Peritoneal dialysis is recommended in acidotic cats with oliguria.

Antidotal therapy

Ethanol is a specific antidote (see above for mechanism) and should be given in any symptomatic case presenting within 24 hours; however, it is probably most effective if given within 12 hours of ingestion. Note: there is no point in giving ethanol to block metabolism if the ethylene glycol has been metabolised. Unfortunately, cases often present late, by which time such antidotal therapy is no longer of use. Management in these cases is supportive. Also, ethanol should not be given to cats with renal failure.

Ethanol regimen

5 ml/kg body weight 20% ethanol in saline, i.v. every 6 hours for 5 doses, then every 8 hours for 4 doses.

Note: In human poisoning cases, once diagnosis has been confirmed by a laboratory, the ethanol given as treatment is given either orally or intravenously. In these cases the recommended doses for 5% and 10% ethanol solutions are identical whatever the route of administration. Therefore, if ethanol in a form suitable for injection is not readily available an equivalent dosing to the above, suitably diluted, could be given orally (ideally by tube direct into the stomach) as an interim measure, e.g. 0.5 ml/kg body weight per hour of a 40% spirit suitably diluted.

Use of ethanol-containing preparations such as methylated spirits or surgical spirits is not recommended as these preparations both contain small quantities of methanol (about 5%).

Bicarbonate regimen

The aim is to keep the urine pH at between 7.5 and 8.0.

(a) With known laboratory analyses:

$$\text{mmol (mEq) of bicarbonate required} = \frac{\text{base deficit} \times 0.5 \times \text{body weight (kg)}}{2}$$

Give slowly over 3–4 hours i.v. Re-check blood gases and assess the clinical status of the animal.

(b) If blood gases are not available, give 0.5–1 mmol/kg body weight i.v. slowly over 30 minutes.

Cats may eat and drink during treatment, although those on ethanol therapy may have CNS depression and may therefore require parenteral or tube feeding.

Calculations

anion gap = $(Na^+ + K^+) - (HCO_3^- + Cl^-)$

osmolar gap = measured osmolality − calculated osmolality

calculated osmolality (mOsmol/kg H_2O) =

$$\frac{(1.86 \times [\text{Na in mmol/L}]) + (\text{urea in mmol/L}) + (\text{glucose in mmol/L})}{0.93}$$

References and further reading

VPIS (London) past cases up to 97/26018.

Clarke P, Henkel K and Swenson C (1997). What is your diagnosis? *Journal of Small Animal Practice* **38**, 433, 450–451.

Dial SM, Thrall MAH and Hamar DW (1994). Comparison of ethanol and 4-methylpyrazole as treatments for ethylene glycol intoxication in cats. *American Journal of Veterinary Research* **55(12)**, 1771–1782.

Dial SM, Thrall MAH and Hamar DW (1994). Efficacy of 4-methylpyrazole for treatment of ethylene glycol intoxication in dogs. *American Journal of Veterinary Research* **55(12)**, 1762–1770.

Grauer GF and Thrall MA (1982). Ethylene glycol (antifreeze) poisoning in the dog and cat. *Journal of the American Hospital Association* **18**, 492–497.

Herd P (1992). Poison – Ethylene Glycol. *In Practice* **14(6)**, 298–299.

Johnson SE et al. (1979). Current status of ethylene glycol toxicity in dogs – a review. *Minnesota Vet* **2**, 32–34.

Proudfoot AT (1993). *Acute Poisoning. Diagnosis and Management* (second edition). Oxford: Butterworth-Heinemann, pp. 120–123.

Rowland J (1987). Incidence of ethylene glycol intoxication in dogs and cats seen at Colorado State University Veterinary Teaching Hospital. *Veterinary and Human Toxicology* **29(1)**, 41–44.

Thrall MA, Grauer GF and Mero KN (1984). Clinicopathologic findings in dogs and cats with ethylene glycol intoxication. *Journal of the American Veterinary Association*, **184(1)**, 37–41.

Ivermectin

Type of product

Ivermectin is an antiparasitic agent and is one of the avermectins. These are natural or semi-natural macrocyclic lactone disaccharides that are fermentation products of *Streptomyces avermitilis* and *Streptomyces cyamogriseus*. Ivermectin is a mixture of about 80% 22,23-dihydroavermectin B_{1a} and 20% 22,23-dihydroavermectin B_{1b}. It is active against mature and immature nematodes and arthropods.

It has veterinary use for the control of mites in cats; migrating heartworm (*Dirofilaria immitis*) larvae in dogs; control of gastrointestinal roundworms and lungworms in horses, ruminants and pigs; Type II ostertagiasis in ruminants; horse bots; some lice and mites on cattle and pigs; warble fly larvae in cattle; and, nasal bots in sheep.

Presentations

Several preparations are available but none specifically for cats, since ivermectin is not officially licensed for feline use in the UK.

In other animals ivermectin may be given orally, subcutaneously or as a pour-on application. Oral preparations may be pastes or liquids and can contain up to 20 mg/dose or up to 1 mg/ml, respectively. Preparations for injection are available at 10 mg/ml strength and pour-on solutions at strengths 5 mg/ml. Some modified release ruminal preparations for cattle are available, designed to release 1.72 g over 135 days.

Occurrence of poisoning incidences

Since 1992 the VPIS London centre has received a small number of enquiries each year regarding ivermectin exposures in cats. One fatality has been reported in a kitten (VPISLn case 97/101602). Several cases involving adult cats that have displayed clinical effects are documented.

Recommended dosage

Ivermectin is not licensed in the UK for use against feline mites, although 'off-license' dosage recommendations are given in some formularies.

Dose regimens: *Octodetes* mites – 200–300 μg/kg body weight s.c. or i.m., repeated after 3 weeks if needed; *Notoedres* mites – 400 μg/kg body weight s.c.

Toxicity

According to the literature:

- A 4 mg oral dose to a cat was associated with severe toxicity with neurological effects.
- Single or multiple oral or subcutaneous doses of 0.2–1.33 mg/kg body weight were reportedly well tolerated in cats.
- 0.2 mg/kg body weight given to cats by s.c. injection resulted in no observable adverse effects.
- 0.4 mg/kg body weight of a preparation intended for cattle given s.c. to cats resulted in dilated pupils, incoordination and hyperaesthesia within 12 hours. The cats recovered within 36 hours.
- A dose of 0.3 mg/kg body weight of a preparation intended for use in cattle given by s.c. injection to a cat resulted in fatality.
- Kittens appear more susceptible to the effects of ivermectin.

In the experience of the VPISLn:

- 2 mg/kg body weight given s.c. to a 1-year-old male neutered cat produced no adverse effects.
- An unknown quantity ingested by a 2-month-old kitten resulted in depression, severe ataxia and death (VPISLn case 97/101602).
- An unknown quantity ingested by a 6-year-old male cat resulted in delayed onset ataxia, incoordination, tremor, dilated pupils, hyperaesthesia and blindness. The animal made gradual recovery over 4 days (VPISLn case 87/24355).

Mechanism of toxicity

Avermectins interfere with parasite nerve transmission by increasing release of the inhibitory neurotransmitter gamma-aminobutyric acid (GABA) from pre-synaptic nerve terminals and enhancing binding to post-synaptic receptors. This leads to the opening of post-synaptic chloride channels causing neuronal hyperpolarisation and depression of neuronal function. They may also act on chloride channels independent of GABA receptors. In invertebrates, where GABA receptors are found in the peripheral nervous system, this causes paralysis, cell dysfunction and death of the animal. In mammals, where GABA receptors are located in the CNS, the result of excess GABA release and post-synaptic binding would be diffuse cerebellar and cerebral cortex dysfunction. However, in mammals avermectins do not readily cross the blood–brain barrier and so toxicity is reduced.

Kinetics and metabolism

Ivermectin appears to be well absorbed following both oral and parental administration with peak levels achieved at about 5.5 hours, and is concentrated in the fat and liver. In high doses it crosses the blood–brain barrier.

Ivermectin is metabolised in the liver into methyl alcohol and monosaccharides and the majority of the metabolites are excreted in the faeces, with only 0.5–2% being excreted in the urine. It is also excreted in the milk of lactating animals.

Clinical effects

Onset of effects is usually within 1–10 hours of oral exposure.

These can be vocalising, disorientation, aggression, anorexia, weakness, lethargy, drowsiness, severe ataxia, blindness, head-pressing, loss of menace reflexes, tremors, dilated pupils and incomplete pupillary response to light.

In more severe cases, bradycardia, hypothermia, respiratory depression, pale mucous membranes, hyporeflexia, retinal atrophy, evidence of multifocal impairment of the thalamus, cerebral cortex and vestibular apparatus, coma and death can occur.

Post-mortem findings

At post-mortem there are no diagnostic lesions observed in ivermectin-poisoned animals. In experimental cases mild pulmonary congestion/oedema and focal CNS haemorrhage were found. However, these findings were not conclusively linked to ivermectin exposure.

Treatment

If exposure was by ingestion and the cat is presented to surgery within 3 hours, induce vomiting or consider gastric lavage, and then administer adsorbents.

Emetics:

(a) Xylazine	Dose:	0.2 mg/kg body weight i.v.; 0.5–1 mg/kg body weight i.m.
(b) Ipecacuanha	Dose:	1–3 ml/kg body weight orally
(c) Soda crystal.		

Adsorbents:

(a) Activated charcoal	Dose:	1–3 g/kg body weight orally
(b) BCK granules®	Dose:	6–18 g orally.

Treatment thereafter is essentially symptomatic and supportive. In particular, the monitoring of electrolytes and fluid balance, blood pressure, heart rate, body temperature, blood gases and respiratory function is advocated.

Contra-indicated drugs

Benzodiazepine use is best avoided in cases of ivermectin toxicity as they also enhance CNS GABAergic activity, owing to ivermectin causing an increased affinity of benzodiazepines for the GABA receptor–chloride channel complex.

Investigations

Plasma levels may be useful in confirming ingestion and toxic exposures.

References and further reading

VPIS (London) past cases up to 97/101602.

Campbell WC and Benz GW (1984). Ivermectin: a review of efficacy and safety. *Journal of Veterinary Pharmacology and Therapeutics* **7**, 1–16.

Hsu WH *et al.* (1989). The safety of ivermectin. *Compendium of Continuing Education: Small Animal Practice* **11(5)**, 584–589.

Kieran P (1987). Toxicity associated with anthelmintics. In *Veterinary Clinical Toxicology, Proceedings No 103* (Proceedings of a conference held at the University of Sydney Australia, 24–28 August, 1987), pp. 443–476.

Lewis DT, Merchant SR and Meer TM (1994). Ivermectin toxicosis in a kitten. *Journal of the American Veterinary Medical Association* **205(4)**, 584–586.

Lovell RA (1990). Ivermectin and piperazine toxicoses in dogs and cats. *Veterinary Clinics of North America: Small Animal Practice* **20(2)**, 453–468.

Paradis M (1998). Ivermectin in small animal dermatology. Part 1. Pharmacology and toxicology. *Compendium on Continuing Education for the Practising Veterinarian* **20(2)**, 193–200.

Roder JD and Stair EL (1998). An overview of ivermectin toxicosis. *Veterinary and Human Toxicology* **40(6)**, 369–370.

Paracetamol

Type of product

Paracetamol is a non-narcotic analgesic with anti-pyretic properties similar to those of aspirin but without anti-inflammatory properties. It has a good safety record in humans when used at recommended dosages.

Presentation

Paracetamol is widely available in the UK as an 'over-the-counter' medication for human use. It is sold under many brand names in both tablet and liquid suspension preparations.

The dose of paracetamol in tablet preparations is variable but the most common strengths encountered are 120 mg and 500 mg. Liquid suspensions are also marketed under a variety of brand names and in varying strengths, though the most commonly encountered strengths are 120 mg/5 ml and 250 mg/5 ml.

Many preparations on the market contain paracetamol in combination with other analgesic drugs, such as aspirin and opioids. Paracetamol may also be found in preparations containing antihistamines, decongestant drugs and caffeine.

Note: In the USA and Canada, paracetamol is called acetaminophen.

Occurrence of poisoning incidences

Since the launch of the VPIS in 1992 paracetamol has been among the most common drugs about which the London centre has been consulted. Until 1996 some 1.9% of enquiries involved paracetamol, with this percentage then rising to 2.5%. Approximately 18% of these enquiries usually involve cats, with 80% involving dogs. The feline cases are usually more serious, with about 25% resulting in fatality. In cats, poisoning most often results from administration by their owners in a misguided attempt to relieve pain, fever and other perceived non-specific ailments.

Recommended dosage

In the UK, the drug is supplied for use in humans only.

There are *no* indications for use of this drug in veterinary medicine. In cats, particularly, its use is potentially very dangerous.

Toxicity

Cats are very sensitive to paracetamol. In particular, they may develop methaemoglobinaemia, haemolytic anaemia, Heinz body formation and hepatic necrosis.

According to the literature:

- Doses of 50–100 mg/kg body weight may cause signs of toxicity to develop.
- Ingestion of one 325 mg tablet resulted in severe toxicosis.
- 173 mg/kg body weight resulted in severe clinical effects. The cat survived after treatment.
- 143 mg/kg body weight proved fatal in one case.
- A single ingestion of 250–500 mg may prove fatal to many cats.
- If one dose has produced no apparent ill effects, a further dose taken within 4–24 hours can be fatal.

In the experience of the VPISLn:

- A dose of 70 mg/kg body weight in one 18-month-old cat produced no clinical effects (VPISLn case 97/3737).
- A dose of 93 mg/kg body weight in an 8-month-old cat produced signs of severe toxicity and death at 12 hours post-ingestion, despite therapy with *N*-acetylcysteine, diuretics, and supportive treatment (VPISLn case 96/2227).
- Administration of single 500 mg tablets in several cats has resulted in severe clinical effects and fatalities, despite prompt antidotal therapy and other treatments (e.g. VPISLn cases 91/45619 and 92/110161).
- A total dose of 1.6 g of paracetamol administered in divided doses over 48 hours to a 1-year-old cat resulted in signs of severe toxicity and death, despite aggressive therapy that included use of *N*-acetylcysteine, ascorbic acid, i.v. Hartmann's solution and whole blood transfusion (VPISLn case 91/45676).
- A dose of 214 mg/kg body weight in one 7-month-old Burmese cat produced severe facial swelling, cyanosis, depression and pyrexia, which responded favourably to administration of *N*-acetylcysteine, cimetidine, steroids and i.v. fluids (VPISLn case 96/121414).

Mechanism of toxicity

Compared with other species, cats have a limited ability to metabolise paracetamol to non-toxic metabolites.

In all species, paracetamol is metabolised in the liver by glucuronidation, sulphation and oxidation. The glucuronide and sulphate conjugates are non-toxic and are excreted in bile and urine. In the metabolism of paracetamol in most species the oxidation pathway is a very minor one, while glucuronidation is the major pathway. However, cats have a restricted ability to conjugate with glucuronic acid as they have low levels of glucuronyl transferase, the enzyme that catalyses the final step of the glucuronidation pathway. Hence, unlike other species except rats, sulphation is the primary route of excretion and the products of the minor oxidation route become more significant.

With increasing paracetamol dosing, the sulphation pathway becomes saturated as, like glucuronidation, it is a capacity-limited process. This results in more paracetamol being metabolised by the restricted glucuronidation route and by oxidation.

At low paracetamol doses some 5% of the drug undergoes oxidation. This pathway, mediated by cytochrome P_{450}, involves N-hydroxylation followed by spontaneous formation of N-acetyl-p-benzoquinoneimine, a highly reactive metabolite. Normally this is conjugated with reduced glutathione, then further metabolised to cysteine and mercaptopuric acid derivatives that are non-toxic and which are excreted in urine. At low dosing this can be an effective and efficient detoxification pathway despite the fact that cats have low glutathione levels.

At higher paracetamol doses when the glucuronidation and sulphation routes are saturated and paracetamol levels in blood and liver rise, the oxidation pathway increases in activity. This results in increased production of N-acetyl-p-benzoquinoneimine, causing glutathione depletion in the liver and subsequently in red blood cells as the detoxification pathway is used. As glutathione becomes depleted the reactive N-acetyl-p-benzoquinoneimine binds covalently with amino acid residues of cellular macromolecules and proteins with subsequent cellular necrosis.

At higher doses paracetamol also inhibits glutathione synthesis, further restricting the capacity of this pathway to produce non-toxic metabolites.

Alternative metabolic pathways also allow accumulation of oxidising metabolites that may induce methaemoglobin formation, Heinz body formation and denaturation of erythrocyte membranes. Heinz bodies are denatured chains of haemoglobin with oxidised sulphydryl groups. They precipitate and migrate towards cell membranes where, perhaps due to alteration of membrane phospholipids, they render cells fragile. Haemolysis and restricted passage of erythrocytes through the microcirculation and spleen may result. Feline haemoglobin is particularly susceptible to oxidative damage as it possesses eight sulphydryl groups per molecule. Methaemoglobinaemia reduces oxygen carrying capacity. It is unclear whether methaemoglobinaemia is directly related to Heinz body formation.

In the presence of glutathione, methaemoglobin will be reduced to haemoglobin. However, when paracetamol levels are high glutathione will be depleted and its synthesis reduced and hence insufficient quantities will be available for this reduction. Methaemoglobin accumulation occurs and as it cannot bind oxygen tissue hypoxia will result. Methaemoglobinaemia further pushes the oxidation dissociation curve to the left, impairing unloading of oxygen further exacerbating the anoxia.

Methaemoglobinaemia normally only occurs when oxidative stress overwhelms erythrocyte capacity.

Hence glutathione availability is crucial in prevention of methaemoglobin and Heinz body formation. It can be seen that increased metabolism of paracetamol via the oxidative pathway is causative of the clinical picture seen in cats following paracetamol administration. The characteristic picture is one of methaemoglobinaemia, cyanosis, anaemia and jaundice. Death usually occurs from progressive methaemoglobinaemia or, more rarely, from severe hepatic necrosis.

Kinetics and metabolism

Paracetamol is rapidly absorbed from the gastrointestinal tract under normal conditions. Clinical manifestations of paracetamol ingestion are normally apparent within 4 hours.

The various metabolic pathways are discussed in the above section on mechanism of toxicity. As the elimination pathways are capacity limited, the plasma half-life is dependent on dose. Experimentally determined half-lives have been recorded at 0.6 hours for a paracetamol dosing of 20 mg/kg body weight, 2.4 hours after 60 mg/kg body weight and 4.8 hours at 120 mg/kg body weight.

At the low dosing of 20 mg/kg body weight the paracetamol is largely metabolised by sulphation, with 5% metabolised by oxidation and 1% by glucuronidation. The sulphation pathway becomes limited at a paracetamol dosing of about 60 mg/kg body weight. At 120 mg/kg body weight sulphation drops to 57%, oxidation rises to 12% and glucuronidation to 16%.

A paracetamol dosing of 60 mg/kg in cats produced a methaemoglobinaemia of 21.7% in 4 hours; 120 mg/kg produced a 45% level.

Clinical effects

Clinical effects usually occur within 4–12 hours.

Prognosis is related to the severity of methaemoglobinaemia that results from the paracetamol ingestion.

Early effects

Within 1–4 hours there may be progressive cyanosis, tachycardia, tachypnoea and dyspnoea, all of which are dependent on the degree of methaemoglobinaemia. Depression, vomiting, inappetence, anorexia, facial (mainly submandibular) and paw oedema, pale mucous membranes, pruritus and hypothermia may also be evident. Rarely, the animals may be hyperthermic. Haematuria, anaemia, and evidence of haemolysis may be present.

Less common effects include ataxia, lethargy, dilated unreactive pupils, nystagmus, photophobia, salivation, lacrimation, abdominal tenderness, hyperaesthesia and twitching.

Later effects

From 2–7 days there may be haemoglobinuria, intravascular haemolysis, icterus and other evidence of liver damage (raised alanine aminotransferase and bilirubin). Coma, convulsions and pulmonary oedema are sometimes reported and are poor prognostic signs. Hepatic necrosis is reported but is not the principal cause of fatality, which in cats is from excessive methaemoglobinaemia.

Renal damage has been reported in paracetamol poisonings in cats. Oliguria is an occasional finding. Death usually occurs between 2 and 6 days post-ingestion.

Laboratory diagnosis

There may be raised alanine aminotransferase, total and direct bilirubin, and elevation of other liver enzymes indicative of icterus. Decreased packed cell volume, methaemoglobinaemia (chocolate blood colour of blood samples) and Heinz body formation may be evident. Haemoglobinuria, proteinuria, and bilirubinuria (dark brown urine colour) have all been reported.

Biochemical abnormalities may take up to 3 weeks to return to normal.

Post-mortem findings

Pulmonary congestion and oedema are sometimes noted. Haemorrhagic congestion, oedema and petechiae of the liver and kidneys are common. Peripheral degenerative changes in the liver include pericholangitis, mononuclear cell infiltrates, bile duct proliferation, biliary stasis and presence of vacuolated hepatocytes. Renal tubular degeneration is occasionally evident.

Unclotted plum/chocolate-coloured blood indicative of methaemoglobinaemia will be present.

Treatment

Treatment is recommended if a dose of 20 mg/kg body weight has been exceeded. Effectively, this means that treatment is needed for ingestion of any commercially available preparation.

If within 2 hours of ingestion, induce vomiting or perform gastric lavage, and then administer adsorbents.

Emetics:

(a)	Xylazine	Dose:	0.2 mg/kg body weight i.v.; 0.5–1 mg/kg body weight i.m.
(b)	Ipecacuanha	Dose:	1–3 ml/kg body weight orally
(c)	Soda crystal.		

Adsorbents:

(a)	Activated charcoal	Dose:	1–3 g/kg body weight orally
(b)	BCK granules®	Dose:	6–18 g orally

Note: Adsorbents should not be given where antidotes are to be administered orally because it may reduce their efficacy.

If the animal is cyanosed, then oxygen should be administered. In addition, there are several antidotal therapies that may be employed.

Antidotal therapy

Probably the most widely used antidote in paracetamol poisoning is N-acetylcysteine because it can significantly reduce the toxicity of the drug by a variety of mechanisms. First, it is a precursor of glutathione. On administration it is hydrolysed to form L-cysteine which provides substrate for glutathione synthesis in red blood cells and the liver. Glutathione cannot be given directly as it is not readily taken up by cells. Second, it acts directly on the reactive metabolite resulting from the cytochrome P_{450} mediated oxidation of paracetamol, N-acetyl-p-benzoquinoneimine, to form an acetylcysteine conjugate, which can be excreted, although this reaction is slow. Third, it is oxidised in the liver to form sulphate, thereby increasing the capacity of the sulphation pathway.

Methionine is a precursor for glutathione and sulphate and has some use. It may be given where N-acetylcysteine is unavailable or used in conjunction with N-acetylcysteine therapy.

Ascorbic acid can be given to reduce methaemoglobin to haemoglobin as it is a good non-enzymatic reductant, although the reaction does occur slowly. There is some evidence to suggest that it may also scavenge N-acetyl-p-benzoquinoneimine before it binds to proteins, possibly reducing it back to paracetamol. This certainly happens in vitro, though there is debate as to whether it happens in vivo. It may be given in combination with the other antidotes.

Administration of sodium sulphate increases the sulphate for conjugation, thereby increasing capacity of the sulphation route of metabolism. It may be used in combination with the other antidotes.

In cases of severe methaemoglobinaemia methylene blue may be used. This drug increases reduction of methaemoglobin. It is reduced to leucomethylene blue by an NADPH-dependent methaemoglobin reductase. The leucomethylene blue then reduces the oxidised haem iron to its normal state. However, it should be used with caution as high doses can themselves cause methaemoglobinaemia or haemolytic anaemia.

Cimetidine is a potent inhibitor of cytochrome P_{450} metabolism in the liver and theoretically administration could result in inhibition of the oxidation pathway. Its efficacy has not been established for paracetamol poisoning cases in cats.

Regimens for antidotes:

(a) N-acetylcysteine   Dose: Either 140 mg/kg body weight orally, wait 6 hours, then 70 mg/kg body weight orally every 6–8 hours for 36 hours or more dependent on the clinical condition of the animal (some sources state it can be given for up to 72 hours) or 280 mg/kg body weight by slow i.v. injection over 6 hours, than 70 mg/kg body weight orally every 6–8 hours for 36 hours or more dependent on the clinical condition of the animal (some sources state it can be given for up to 72 hours).

Note: The second method should be employed if adsorbents have previously been given.

(b) Methionine   Dose: 70 mg/kg body weight orally every 6–8 hours, up to 24 hours.

Note: If adsorbents have previously been given, a 6-hour period should elapse before administration is started.

(c) Ascorbic acid   Dose: 30–40 mg/kg body weight i.v. every 6–8 hours until no cyanosis is present.

(d) Sodium sulphate   Dose: 1.6% solution; 50 mg/kg body weight i.v. every 4 hours, up to 24 hours.

(e) Methylene blue   Dose: 1–5 mg/kg body weight by slow intravenous injection.

(f) Cimetidine   Dose: 2.5–5 mg/kg body weight i.v., i.m. or orally two–three times daily.

Other care

Management is otherwise symptomatic and supportive, with particular care being taken to ensure adequate hydration and maintenance of body temperature. Use of heat pads or other warming methods have been required in some cases.

Urea, electrolytes and blood gases should be checked if possible and corrected where necessary. The animal should also be monitored for evidence of liver damage, anaemia and haemolysis. If there is evidence of severe haemolysis, significant decrease in packed cell volume, or severe anaemia, then whole blood transfusions may be required.

It is recommended that blood counts are monitored for at least 1 week post-therapy.

References and further reading

VPIS (London) past cases up to 97/11295.

Brown F (1985). Paracetamol poisoning in cats. *Veterinary Record* 116, 275.

Davis MR (1985). Paracetamol poisoning in a cat. *Veterinary Record* 116, 223.

Hjelle JJ and Grauer GF (1986). Acetaminophen-induced toxicosis in dogs and cats. *Journal of the American Veterinary Medical Association* 188(7), 742–746.

Hornfeldt CS (1992). Distinction made between toxicoses caused by acetaminophen and non-steroidal anti-inflammatory drugs. *Journal of the American Veterinary Medical Association* 201(9), 1318–1319.

Ilkiw JE and Ratcliffe RC (1987). Paracetamol toxicity in a cat. *Australian Veterinary Journal* 64(8), 245–247.

Judson DG (1985). Paracetamol poisoning in cats. *Veterinary Record* 116, 355.

Kolf-Clauw M and Keck G (1994). Paracetamol poisoning in dogs and cats. *European Journal of Companion Animal Practice* 4, 85–92.

Kore AM (1997). Over-the-counter analgesic drug toxicoses in small animals. *Veterinary Medicine* 92(2), 158–165.

Lorenzana RM (1985). Paracetamol poisoning in cats. *Veterinary Record* 117, 135.

Lugten PC (1985). Paracetamol poisoning in cats. *Veterinary Record* 116, 424.

Malley AD (1987). Paracetamol poisoning in a cat. *Veterinary Record* 121, 528.

Marcella KL (1983). Acetaminophen poisoning in cats and man. *Journal of the American Veterinary Medical Association* 183(8), 836.

Mayer S (1991). Poison – Paracetamol. *In Practice* 13(1), 37.

Nicol RG (1981). Treatment of paracetamol poisoning in cats. *Veterinary Record* 109, 291.

Prasuhn LW (1983). Tylenol poisoning in the cat. *Journal of the American Veterinary Medical Association* 182(1), 4–5.

Savides MC et al. (1984). The toxicity and biotransformation of single doses of acetaminophen in dogs and cats. *Toxicology and Applied Pharmacology* 74, 26–34.

Thursby-Pelham C (1996). Peculiar drug poisonings in pets. *In Practice* 18(10), 478–487.

Villar D, Buck WB and Gonzalez JM (1998). Ibuprofen, aspirin and acetaminophen toxicosis and treatment in dogs and cats. *Veterinary and Human Toxicology* 40(3), 156–161.

Walker PD (1985). Paracetamol poisoning in cats. *Veterinary Record* 116, 301.

Piperazine

Type of product

Piperazine is an anthelmintic used for the treatment of roundworms in cats, dogs, horses, pigs and poultry.

Presentation

Piperazine is commonly available in tablet and syrup formulations. Paste and powder formulations for oral administration are also available. Preparations use a variety of piperazine salts, but commonly the citrate, phosphate, hydrate or adipate.

Strengths of citrate-based tablet preparations are 125 mg, 220 mg, 275 mg, and 500 mg; syrup preparations 80 mg/ml or 100 mg/ml and pastes 250 mg/g. Strengths of phosphate-based tablet preparations are 104 mg and 416 mg. Strength of the hydrate-based syrup preparation is 58 mg/ml. Strength of the adipate-based tablet preparation is 500 mg.

A measure of 100 mg of piperazine hydrate is equivalent to:

- 120 mg piperazine adipate
- 125 mg piperazine citrate
- 104 mg piperazine phosphate.

There are a few preparations combining piperazine with other anthelmintics, such as dichlorophen.

Occurrence of poisoning incidences

Since the launch of the VPIS, between five and 25 enquiries per year have been received regarding piperazine ingestion or administration to cats and dogs. Over 80% of the enquiries concern cats. Four cases with a fatal outcome are documented, one involving a dichlorophen combination preparation, but in all these cases the dose ingested was unknown.

Recommended dosage

This is 80–100 mg/kg body weight orally for *Toxocara* or *Toxascaris* infections to a maximum of 250 mg in animals less than 2.5 kg body weight; 120–240 mg/kg body weight orally for *Uncinaria* or *Ancylostoma* infections.

Use is contra-indicated in animals with renal impairment.

Toxicity

Piperazine is of relatively low toxicity, but may cause transient neurotoxicity in some individuals. It is not known why some individuals are susceptible to piperazine toxicity.

According to the literature:

- Doses of >800 mg/kg body weight are likely to produce neurotoxicity.
- Clinical effects have been seen at therapeutic doses.

In the experience of the VPISLn:

- A dose of 76 mg/kg body weight produced transient ataxia and hyperaesthesia in a 7-year-old Burmese cat. The animal made a slow recovery.

Mechanism of toxicity

Piperazine blocks acetylcholine and acts as a GABA agonist, causing hyperpolarisation of parasite muscle cells. This temporarily paralyses the target worm causing its release from the gut wall and subsequent expulsion from the body in the faeces. The toxic effects appear to be due to the anticholinergic actions of the drug, but possibly also its GABA-ergic effects.

Clinical effects

Clinical effects usually occur within 24 hours but may have a duration of 2–4 days.

Commonly reported effects are vomiting, diarrhoea, anorexia, dilated pupils, weakness, ataxia, lethargy, incoordination, tremor, hyperaesthesia, hyperventilation and convulsions.

Treatment

Treatment is recommended for ingestions >240 mg/kg body weight for hydrate, >288 mg/kg body weight for adipate, >300 mg/kg body weight for citrate and >250 mg/kg body weight for phosphate.

Note: These doses are given only as a guide; some animals may exhibit toxicity at lower doses.

If within 2 hours of ingestion, induce vomiting or perform gastric lavage, and then administer adsorbents.

Emetics:

(a) Xylazine	Dose:	0.2 mg/kg body weight i.v.; 0.5–1 mg/kg body weight i.m.
(b) Ipecacuanha	Dose:	1–3 ml/kg body weight orally
(c) Soda crystal.		

Adsorbents:

(a) Activated charcoal	Dose:	1–3 g/kg body weight orally
(b) BCK granules®	Dose:	6–18 g orally.

Treatment is symptomatic and supportive. Keeping the animal in a quiet, dark place may be of benefit. There is no specific antidote.

Diazepam may be used for sedation or the control of convulsions. Dose: 0.5 mg/kg body weight i.v. repeated every 10 minutes up to three times to effect.

References and further reading

VPIS (London) past cases up to 97/116526.

Darke PGG (1987). Piperazine toxicity. *Veterinary Record* **120**, 507.

Goddard PC and Johnston AM (1986). Piperazine toxicity in a kitten. *Veterinary Record* **119(25–26)**, 625.

Gray AK and Millar JE (1987). Piperazine toxicity in a kitten. *Veterinary Record* **120(2)**, 48.

Hartigan PJ (1987). Piperazine toxicity. *Veterinary Record* **120(3)**, 70.

Howroyd PC (1984). Side effects from piperazine. *Veterinary Record* **115(6)**, 136.

Lovell RA (1990). Ivermectin and piperazine toxicoses in dogs and cats. *Veterinary Clinics of North America: Small Animal Practice* **20 (2)**, 453–468.

Swift BJ (1984). Side effects from piperazine? *Veterinary Record* **114(25)**, 623.

Pyrethrins and pyrethroids

Type of product

Pyrethrins (jasmolin I and II, cinerin I and II, pyrethrin I and II) are naturally occurring esters of chrysanthemic acid and pyrethric acid, which are extracted from the flowers of *Chrysanthemum cinerariaefolium*.

Pyrethroids (allethrin, alphacypermethrin, bioresmethrin, cypermethrin, deltamethrin, fenvalerate, permethrin, phenothrin, resmethrin, tetramethrin) are synthetic pyrethrins.

Pyrethrins and pyrethroids are used as insecticides for the treatment of ectoparasitic infestation. They are used in cats, dogs, sheep, cattle, poultry, horses, goats and humans.

Presentation

Pyrethroids and pyrethrins are used on cats for the control of fleas, biting flies and lice. Preparations are available as dusting powders, shampoos and sprays.

Note that cats may also be exposed to agrochemical preparations not designed for veterinary use. Some of these may contain other constituents, including other insecticides and solvents. Piperonyl butoxide is often added to the insecticide preparations as a synergist (it delays the metabolism of the insecticide and increases the toxicity).

Occurrence of poisoning incidences

Since 1992 the London centre of the VPIS has received between 10 and 50 enquiries per annum regarding pyrethroids and pyrethrins in animals. Approximately 65% of these involve cats. Intoxication either occurs as a result of ingestion of products or through over-zealous application of insecticide preparations to the coats of the cats. Many of the feline cases arise as a result of dermal application of products intended for use in dogs. These contain similar ingredients as the feline products but often in higher concentrations.

Toxicity may result from self-grooming of treated fur. Occasionally, toxicity may arise from animals being in close association with or grooming treated animals.

Recommended dosage

This varies with the individual preparation.

Toxicity

In the experience of the VPISLn:

- A 1-year-old female domestic short-haired cat consumed a permethrin-containing insecticide. Within 2 hours the cat had tachycardia, salivation, hyperpnoea, ataxia, tremors and convulsions. The cat was given atropine and supportive care and the effects resolved after 9 hours (VPISLn case 92/68353).
- A three-and-a-half-year-old 4.5 kg cat was accidentally treated with a permethrin-based insecticide intended for canine use. The animal developed convulsions, tachycardia, hyperaesthesia, dilated pupils and mild trismus. The cat was given diazepam, washed and then collared to prevent grooming, and given supportive care and a low-fat diet. The animal had recovered fully within 48 hours (VPISLn case 95/164979).
- A 4 kg cat was treated with a flea spray containing permethrin and piperonyl butoxide. Within 5 hours the animal had profuse salivation, hyperaesthesia and convulsions. The animal died, despite supportive care (VPISLn case 94/152472)

Mechanism of toxicity

The toxic effects of pyrethroids and pyrethrins are due to alteration of the kinetics of voltage-dependent sodium channels in nerve membranes, which causes repetitive discharges or membrane depolarisation. Some pyrethroids may also inhibit gamma aminobutyric acid (GABA) receptors. This inhibits the $GABA_A$-receptor mediated chloride ion influx, the physiological function of which is to induce presynaptic inhibition. Loss of this inhibition can lead to hyperexcitability of nervous tissue and may be the mechanism by which these compounds produce convulsions.

In mammals pyrethrins and pyrethroids are rapidly biotransformed and detoxified by ester hydrolysis or oxidation. As a result, these compounds are of relatively low toxicity in mammals. Also, the activity of these compounds on sodium channels is negatively correlated to temperature and the greater toxicity in insects may also be an effect of the lower body temperature of insects.

Intoxication may occur in individual cats. Cats are more susceptible to toxicity than dogs. Toxicity is more common in young cats (<4 years, particularly <1 year), but the reason for this is unclear. Dermal exposure is the most common route in cats. There is probably some dermal absorption but there may be some ingestion of the chemical due to grooming. Occasionally, toxicity may arise from animals being in close association with or grooming treated animals.

The feline liver is relatively inefficient at glucuronide conjugation. This leads to slow excretion and accumulation of metabolites and may be the reason for the common occurrence of toxicity in cats. Pyrethroids and pyrethrins are lipophilic and if repeatedly administered can accumulate in fatty tissues.

Note: Non-specific plasma esterases are important for detoxification of most pyrethroids and pyrethrins (except allethrin and pyrethrum). Organophosphorous insecticides inhibit these enzymes and simultaneous exposure to these insecticides will increase the toxicity of pyrethrins and pyrethroids.

Clinical effects

Onset usually occurs within 1–3 hours, sometimes up to 12 hours, duration 1–3 days.

Note: Simultaneous exposure to organophosphate insecticides may increase the toxicity of pyrethroids and pyrethrins (see above). Piperonyl butoxide, often added as a synergist to delay metabolism and increase toxicity in insects, produces effects similar to that of pyrethrins and pyrethroids.

Vomiting, diarrhoea, salivation, ataxia, tremor, incoordination, twitching, dilated pupils, tachycardia, hyperexcitibility, hyperaesthesia, thirst, pyrexia, hyperpnoea, muscle weakness and fasciculations and convulsions have all been reported. Respiratory distress, probably due to weakness of respiratory muscles, may occur.

Some compounds cause paraesthesia, for example shaking of feet when they are dry.

Treatment

If within 2 hours of ingestion, induce vomiting or perform gastric lavage, and then administer adsorbents.

Emetics:

(a) Xylazine	Dose:	0.2 mg/kg body weight i.v.; 0.5–1 mg/kg body weight i.m.
(b) Ipecacuanha	Dose:	1–3 ml/kg body weight orally
(c) Soda crystal.		

Adsorbents:

(a) Activated charcoal	Dose:	1–3 g/kg body weight orally
(b) BCK granules®	Dose:	6–18 g orally.

Treatment is essentially symptomatic and supportive. If the exposure is dermal, the cat should be washed with lukewarm water and detergent. The use of very warm water should be avoided as this increases dermal perfusion and may result in increased dermal absorption. Copious amounts of detergent should be used because pyrethrins and pyrethroids are not soluble in water.

Diazepam or pentobarbitone may be used to control twitching, fasciculation or convulsions. Diazepam dose: 0.5 mg/kg body weight i.v. repeated every 10 minutes up to three times if needed; Pentobarbitone dose: 3–15 mg/kg body weight by slow intravenous infusion.

Care should be taken to maintain hydration and body temperature. Atropine may be given for hypersalivation. If temperature rises due to muscle fasciculation, cerebral oedema may result, which can lead to continued convulsions.

Fatty foods should not be given because these will enhance absorption.

References and further reading

VPIS (London) past cases up to 97/129997 (permethrin), 97/134900 (pyrethroids).

Nicholson SS (1995). Toxicity of insecticides and skin care products of botanical origin. *Veterinary Dermatology* **6(3)**, 139–143.

Powers KA *et al.* (1988). An evaluation of the acute toxicity of an a insecticidal spray containing linalol, D-limonene and piperonyl butoxide applied topically to domestic cats. *Veterinary and Human Toxicology* **30(3)**, 206–210.

Valentine WM (1990). Pyrethrin and pyrethroid insecticides. *Veterinary Clinics of North America: Small Animal Practice* **20(2)**, 375–382.

Whittem T (1995). Pyrethrin and pyrethroid insecticide intoxication in cats. *The Compendium* **17(4)**, 489–492.

Benzodiazepines

Type of product

Benzodiazepines are mainly used as hypnotics/sedatives, but also have use as anxiolytics, anticonvulsants and premedicants. There are 16 available benzodiazepines in the UK. Of these, five are listed in the veterinary formularies for use in veterinary practice: alprazolam, clonazepam, clorazepate, diazepam and midazolam.

Presentation

The benzodiazepines are available in tablet, capsule, liquid and injectable forms at a variety of strengths. Some of the benzodiazepines intended for human use are also available as rectal tubes and suppositories.

Alprazolam	250 μg, 500 μg tablets
Bromazepam	1.5 mg, 3 mg tablets
Chlordiazepoxide	5 mg, 10 mg, 25 mg tablets; 5 mg, 10 mg capsules
Clobazam	10 mg tablets
Clonazepam	0.5 mg, 2 mg tablets; 1 mg/ml injection
Clorazepate	7.5 mg, 15 mg tablets
Diazepam	2 mg, 5 mg, 10 mg tablets; 2 mg/5 ml, 5 mg/5 ml oral solutions; 5 mg/ml injection; 10 mg suppository; 2 mg/ml, 4 mg/ml rectal tubes
Flunitrazepam	1 mg tablets
Flurazepam	15 mg, 30 mg tablets
Loprazolam	1 mg tablets
Lorazepam	1 mg, 4 mg tablets; 4 mg/ml injection
Lormetazepam	0.5 mg, 1 mg tablets
Midazolam	1 mg/ml, 2 mg/ml, 5 mg/ml injection
Nitrazepam	5 mg tablets; 2.5 mg/5 ml oral solution
Oxazepam	10 mg, 15 mg, 30 mg tablets
Temazepam	10 mg, 20 mg tablets; 10 mg, 15 mg, 20 mg, 30 mg capsules; 10 mg/5 ml oral elixir.

Occurrence of poisoning incidences

Since 1992 the VPIS has received between 15 and 40 enquiries per annum regarding exposure of companion animals to benzodiazepine drugs. Cases involving dogs predominate and almost all involve pets inadvertently consuming their owners' medication. Nitrazepam, temazepam and diazepam are those that have been frequently consumed. No fatal cases have been reported.

Recommended dosage

Diazepam

Status epilepticus: 0.5 mg/kg body weight i.v. bolus, repeat after 10 minutes if necessary.

Anaesthetic premedicant/sedative: 0.1–0.25 mg/kg body weight i.v.

Anxiolytic (cats): 0.22 mg–2 mg/kg body weight orally, 8 hourly.

Appetite stimulant (cats): 0.5–1 mg/kg body weight i.v.

Spraying (cats): 1.25–2.5 mg/cat 8–12 hourly.

Scotty cramp (dogs): 0.5–2 mg/kg body weight i.v., then orally every 8 hours.

Alprazolam

Anxiety (cats): 0.125–0.25 mg/cat, 2–3 times daily.

Clonazepam

Status epilepticus (dogs): 50–200 μg/kg body weight i.v.

Clorazepate

Anxiety: 0.55–2.2 mg/kg body weight 1–2 times daily

Midazolam

Sedation: 66–200 μg/kg body weight i.v.

Toxicity

Benzodiazepines are of low toxicity, both in therapy and in overdose. In therapeutic doses, both the cardiovascular and respiratory effects are minimal. Muscle relaxation may occur, but this is seldom a problem in dogs and cats. Benzodiazepines can cause disinhibition, leading to paradoxical hyperactivity or aggression. In debilitated animals or in overdose, respiratory depression may become clinically significant and necessitate ventilation.

The long-term use of benzodiazepines has been associated with liver damage in both dogs and cats.

According to the literature:

- The Centre National d'Informations Toxicologiques Vétérinaraires (CNITV) followed up cases of benzodiazepine poisoning in animals between 1991 and 1994. There were 463 calls relating to dogs and 49 to cats. The common clinical effects were ataxia, hyperactivity, muscle tremors and coma. They postulated that, because the half-lives for many benzodiazepines are shorter in dogs, they are less toxic. No deaths were reported (Bertini *et al.*, 1995).

- Two dogs, deliberately poisoned, were presented with lethargy leading to coma, tonic and clonic convulsions with extensor rigidity and pulmonary haemorrhage. Both animals were euthanased. *Flurazepam* was detected in the urine of one dog (Beier and Bischoff, 1997).
- Eleven cases of fulminant hepatic failure were reported in cats. Clinical signs developed within 5–11 days of initial oral treatment with *diazepam*. Dosage ranged from 1 mg daily to 2.5 mg twice daily. Eight cats died 7–15 days after initial treatment. The authors considered the hepatotoxicosis idiosyncratic as all but one cat were treated within the established dosage range (Center *et al.*, 1996).
- The oral LD_{50} for *lorazepam* in dogs is >2 g/kg body weight.
- The oral LD_{50} for *temazepam* in dogs is quoted as 3.62 g/kg body weight.
- The oral LD_{50} for *flurazepam* in cats is quoted as 250 mg/kg body weight.
- The parenteral LD_{50} for *diazepam* in dogs is >800 mg/kg body weight.

In the experience of the VPISLn:

- No fatal cases reported.
- A dose of 8.3 mg/kg body weight of *clonazepam* in a dog caused hyperaesthesia, salivation, ataxia and tremors (VPISLn case 92/84883).
- 1 mg/kg body weight of *diazepam* in a dog caused respiratory depression (VPISLn case 92/53570).
- Doses of *diazepam* up to 22 mg/kg body weight in dogs caused ataxia and lethargy only.
- *Diazepam* at a dosing of 40 mg/kg body weight in one dog caused prolonged sedation, hypotension and hypothermia (VPISLn case 94/101681).
- 2.2 mg/kg of *nitrazepam* in a dog caused drowsiness, salivation and severe ataxia (VPISLn case 95/100903). Higher doses in other animals produced drowsiness only.
- A *temazepam* dose of 1.3 mg/kg body weight in a dog produced drowsiness in one case (VPISLn case 93/80648), whereas doses up to 5.5 mg/kg in other animals produced no effects.
- 40 mg/kg body weight of *temazepam* in one dog produced drowsiness only (VPISLn case 96/22554).

Mechanism of toxicity

Benzodiazepines act by enhancing the effect of the inhibitory neurotransmitter gamma-amino-butyric-acid (GABA). GABA binds to a specific receptor complex located in the CNS. This causes chloride ions to move from the extracellular to the intracellular space. Increased flow of chloride ions leads to hyperpolarisation of the cell and inhibition. This receptor complex also contains binding sites for benzodiazepines, enhancing the effect of GABA. An overdose will increase this inhibition, resulting in greater sedation.

Kinetics and metabolism

Benzodiazepines are rapidly absorbed from the gastrointestinal tract. They are metabolised in the liver, some to pharmacolgically active intermediates and are excreted via the kidneys. Benzodiazepines are usually classed as short-, intermediate- or long-acting, dependent on their half-lives.

Clinical effects

Clinical effects usually occur between 30 minutes and 2 hours following ingestion.

Commonly occurring effects include ataxia, drowsiness, muscle tremors, vomiting, hypothermia and coma. In severe cases respiratory depression may be seen. Paradoxically, there may be hyperaesthesia, hypersalivation, agitation, aggressiveness, hyperactivity and hyperthermia.

Chronic exposures may result in liver damage, the initial signs of which are non-specific and include variable anorexia, vomiting, lethargy, dehydration, hypothermia and jaundice.

Treatment

If the animal presents to surgery within 2 hours of ingestion, then adsorbents should be given. For massive overdose gastric lavage may be considered as may use of emetics, provided the animal is not too drowsy.

Adsorbents:

(a) Activated charcoal	Dose:	2 g/kg body weight orally
(b) BCK granules®	Dose:	6–18 g orally 2–3 times daily.

Emetics:

(a) Apomorphine	Dose:	0.05 mg/kg body weight i.v. or i.m.; 0.1 mg/kg body weight s.c.
(b) Xylazine	Dose:	0.2 mg/kg body weight i.v.; 0.5–1 mg/kg body weight i.m. or s.c.
(c) Ipecacuanha	Dose:	1–2 ml/kg body weight (maximum 20 ml) orally
(d) Soda crystal.		

Note: Apomorphine use is contra-indicated in cats.

The animal should be observed for a minimum of 4 hours post-ingestion. Management is essentially symptomatic and supportive. Cooling/warming measures should be instituted as appropriate. In severe cases, ventilation may be necessary.

A specific benzodiazepine receptor antagonist called flumazenil is available. In human medicine it is licensed for reversal of sedative effects of benzodiazepines in anaesthetic, intensive care and diagnostic procedures only. Its use in animals has, to date, been limited. Doses of 0.3–30 mg/kg body weight have been used experimentally in mice and cats to successfully antagonise the central effects of some benzodiazepine agents. A suggested dose for dogs and cats is 0.1–0.2 mg/kg body weight given i.v., i.m. or s.c.

In cases of suspected liver damage following chronic exposures, liver function tests should be carried out.

References and further reading

VPIS (London) past cases up to 98/154230.

Bertini S et al. (1995). Benzodiazepine poisoning in companion animals. *Veterinary and Human Toxicology* **37**(6), 559–562.

Beier E and Bischoff K (1997). Flurazepam toxicosis in two dogs. *Veterinary and Human Toxicology* **39**(6), 352–354.

Center SA et al. (1996). Fulminant hepatic failure associated with oral administration of diazepam in 11 cats. *Journal of the American Veterinary Medical Association* **209**(3), 618–625.

Bogden RN and Goa KL (1991). Flumazenil, a reappraisal of its pharmacological properties and therapeutic efficacy as a benzodiazepine antagonist. *Drugs* **42**, 1061–1089.

Petroleum distillates / White spirit / Kerosene

Type of product

Petroleum distillates are usually complex chemical mixtures derived from the distillation of crude oil. They include both aliphatic and aromatic hydrocarbons.

White spirit is a mixture of aliphatic hydrocarbons C_9–C_{12}, naphthalene and higher aromatics. Kerosene is a mixture of aliphatic hydrocarbons C_9–C_{16}, olefins and aromatics, including naphthalene.

Presentation

They are usually liquid and have characteristic strong odours. Examples are petrol, paraffin, diesel, solvents for paints (especially gloss paints), varnishes, glues, glass cleaners, lamp oils, barbecue lighter fluids and sometimes as a liquid vehicle for pesticides, wood preservatives, and industrial chemicals.

White spirit is usually a colourless volatile liquid commonly found in the home as a paintbrush cleaner. Turpentine substitute is white spirit.

Occurrence of poisoning incidences

Since 1992 the London centre of the VPIS has received between 20 and 60 enquiries per annum regarding petroleum distillate or white spirit exposures in cats and dogs. Some 75% of these enquiries involve white spirit or turpentine substitute, as these are the most likely products to be found in the home. Three fatal cases are documented, two in cats and one in a dog.

Toxicity

According to the literature:

- Aspiration of as little as 5 ml of refined petroleum distillates may result in fatal aspiration pneumonia.

In the experience of VPISLn:

- A 3 kg domestic short-haired cat had access to the spilled contents of a large bottle of white spirit for some hours. It was assumed the animal had inhaled the vapours and had also walked through the spill. Oral exposure had occurred through grooming. The animal had severe skin burns, abdominal tenderness, severe buccal irritation and gradually deteriorating respiratory function over 2 days. Despite aggressive therapy with analgesics, fluids and antibiotics the animal died. Cause of death was attributed to severe pulmonary oedema (VPISLn case 92/ 88577). A similar exposure and outcome occurred in another 4.5 kg cat (VPISLn case 94/109826).

• A 13-year-old Setter drank an unknown quantity of white spirit from a spilled 1 litre container whilst unminded. The animal was found collapsed and distressed, with severe buccal irritation, panting, wheezing, and ataxia. The animal was sedated, and given steroids, antibiotics and adsorbents but was later euthanased as no significant improvement was apparent (VPISLn case 97/130559).

Mechanism of toxicity

Petroleum distillates and white spirit are generally irritant to skin and mucous membranes, but also may cause CNS depression if inhaled at high concentrations or for prolonged periods or if ingested in large quantities.

The most severe clinical problems associated with exposure are due to aspiration pneumonia. The more volatile or highly refined the petroleum distillate mixture, the greater the risk of aspiration and development of pulmonary oedema. This is owing to the low surface tension, which allows widespread diffusion into the lungs even when small quantities of fluid are involved.

Clinical effects

Onset of effects is usually between 1 and 8 hours post-exposure.

Ingestion or oral exposure following grooming after dermal exposure may cause salivation, severe and protracted vomiting, local irritation and ulceration of the mouth and throat, abdominal tenderness, diarrhoea, inappetence and anorexia.

Signs of systemic toxicity include tachycardia, ataxia, tremor, weakness, excitability and agitation. Convulsions, tachypnoea, hyperaesthesia and pyrexia are reported for more severe exposures.

Aspiration pneumonia is an occasional complication of ingestion where coughing or vomiting has occurred. It also occurs following inhalation. Clinical effects include coughing, fever, dyspnoea, cyanosis and, in severe cases, CNS depression and pulmonary oedema.

Petroleum distillates are irritant to skin and eyes. Blisters, inflammation and burns have been reported following dermal exposures and corneal damage has occurred when such compounds come into contact with eyes.

Post-mortem findings

The most common finding is that of severe pulmonary oedema. The lungs are usually congested. Hepatic fatty change and renal cell degeneration and necrosis are occasional findings.

Treatment

Use of emetics and gastric lavage is contraindicated owing to the risk of aspiration. Adsorbents are of limited benefit. They reportedly bind aromatic distillates and longer chain aliphatic hydrocarbons and therefore may help to reduce absorption of distillate mixtures such as kerosene.

Adsorbents:

(a) Activated charcoal	Dose:	2 g/kg body weight orally
(b) BCK granules®	Dose:	6–18 g orally.

Oral fluids should be encouraged.

Where dermal exposure has occurred, the animal should be thoroughly washed. Petroleum distillates are not very miscible with water so *non-solvent*-based detergents or commercially available hand degreasers, e.g. Swarfega®, may need to be employed. Where possible the animal should be collared to prevent further grooming and further ingestion of the distillate.

Contaminated eyes should be irrigated with water or saline, and then stained with fluorescein and examined for corneal injury.

Treatment thereafter is symptomatic and supportive. Bland diets are recommended if there is evidence of severe buccal irritation. Care should be taken to ensure adequate hydration and nutrition. Atropine may be given for excessive salivation.

An observation period of 12 hours is recommended.

The animal should be assessed for respiratory effects. Aspiration pneumonia requires conventional therapy, with oxygen supplementation and cage rest. In severe cases positive end-expiratory pressure ventilation (PEEP) may be considered, though it should be used with caution as pneumomediastinum and pneumothorax are potential complications.

The use of antibiotics to prevent secondary lung infections is recommended.

References

VPIS (London) past cases up to 97/130559.

Dorman DC (1990). Petroleum distillates and turpentine. *Veterinary Clinics of North America: Small Animal Practice* **20(2)**, 505–513.

Owens JG and Dorman DC (1997). Common household hazards for small animals. *Veterinary Medicine* **92(2)**, 140–148.

Poinsettia / *Euphorbia pulcherrima*

The plant

The common name for *Euphorbia pulcherrima* is poinsettia. The plant belongs to the Euphorbiaceae family.

These are largely encountered as ornamental plants. They may grow from 30–40 cm in height, and have bright red-coloured bracts, though some may be pink or off-white-coloured.

Occurrence of poisoning incidences

Since the launch of the VPIS the centre in London has received a small number of enquiries each year regarding ingestion of Poinsettia by both cats and dogs. In most cases, the animals remain asymptomatic. Ingestion or exposure is common in winter months, when the plant bears red leaves and is used as a festive decoration.

Toxicity

This plant is considered of low toxicity.

According to the literature:

- One case with a fatal outcome is described where a cat developed severe gastrointestinal upset, pyrexia and died after consuming leaves from a poinsettia plant.

In the experience of the VPISLn:

- Ingestion usually results in mild gastrointestinal effects only.
- In one case, a Burmese kitten who ate a large leaf showed severe buccal irritation and endoscopy revealed severe oesophageal irritation (VPISLn case 96/191501).

Mechanism of toxicity

The plant, like most Euphorbia species, contains diterpene esters, but concentrations in poinsettia are very low compared to other species. The principal effects of ingestion would be irritant ones.

Clinical effects

These can be vomiting, salivation, diarrhoea, abdominal tenderness and, rarely, pyrexia.

Treatment

Gastric decontamination using gastric lavage, emesis or adsorbents is not necessary unless huge amounts of plant material have been ingested.

Management should otherwise be supportive, particularly ensuring that the animal is well hydrated.

Reference

VPIS (London) past cases up to 97/43709.

Silica gel

Type of product

Silica gel is a commonly used desiccant.

Presentation

Small packets of silica gel are often found in the packaging of electrical goods, shoes, cameras and containers for drugs.

Occurrence of poisoning incidences

Every year the VPIS receives numerous enquiries abut the potential toxicity of silica gel to domestic pets. In the cases reported, no serious clinical effects have resulted in either cats or dogs.

Toxicity

Silica gel is inert and not toxic; however the packets are often misleadingly labelled with a skull and cross bones and the words 'Do not eat'. As a result, silica gel is a frequent cause of unnecessary concern.

Clinical effects

None are anticipated.

Treatment

No treatment is necessary, even for very substantial ingestions.

Reference

VPIS (London) past cases up to 98/154124.

Thermometers

Type of product

Instruments for the measurement of temperature, both clinical thermometers for body temperature measurement and thermometers for determining ambient temperature, are available.

Presentation

They usually consist of a glass tube with a bulbous end containing a liquid, which changes in volume depending on the temperature.

Occurrence of poisoning incidences

The VPIS receives a small number of enquiries each year regarding ingestion of mercury thermometers by dogs. No serious cases have arisen.

Toxicity

Clinical thermometers contain about 1 g of elemental mercury (approximately 0.1 ml). Mercury in this form is not absorbed from the gut to any great extent, therefore systemic toxicity is unlikely to occur from ingestion of the contents of clinical thermometers.

Thermometers for the measurement of ambient temperature (both indoor and outdoor) usually contain 0.3–0.5 ml of triethyl phosphate, toluene, xylene or an alcohol. The quantity of harmful substances in these thermometers is not significant.

Clinical effects

Ingestion of a mercury-containing thermometer may cause mild gastrointestinal irritation until all the mercury is passed in the faeces.

Treatment

No treatment is necessary. An X-ray may reveal mercury droplets in the gut following ingestion of a mercury-containing thermometer but no treatment is required.

Often the only real risk following ingestion of a thermometer is from the glass. The mouth should be checked for cuts and any glass fragments removed.

Reference

VPIS (London) past cases up to 98/85762.

Allopurinol

Type of product

Allopurinol is a xanthine oxidase inhibitor with veterinary use in the prophylactic management of recurrent uric acid uroliths and hyperuricosuric calcium oxalate urolithiasis. It has human use in prophylactic management of idiopathic gout and prevention of calcium oxalate and uric acid renal stones.

Presentation

Allopurinol is widely available in the UK as a prescription medicine for both veterinary and human use. Various proprietary preparations are available. Most preparations are in tablet form and are of 100 mg or 300 mg strength.

Occurrence of poisoning incidences

Since the launch of the VPIS in 1992 there have been up to 10 enquiries per year concerning allopurinol ingestion by dogs. No fatal cases have occurred and most of the animals involved remained asymptomatic. In the majority of cases the animals consumed tablets intended for use by their owners, rather than being accidentally overdosed on their own medication.

Recommended dosage

The recommended dose for dogs is 10 mg/kg body weight orally every 8 hours for one month, followed by 10–20 mg/kg body weight orally per day.

Toxicity

According to the literature:

- Dogs receiving doses in excess of 200 mg/kg body weight per day for 1 year developed renal xanthine deposits.
- Daily doses of 2–4 g have been survived in dogs.

In the experience of the VPISLn:

- Acute doses as high as 750 mg/kg body weight have not caused any clinical effects.
- Delayed diarrhoea and polydipsia was linked to ingestion of 15 g by a small dog (VPISLn case 92/102518).
- 4 g reportedly caused a period of excitability in a Dalmatian (VPISLn case 96/111279).

Mechanism of toxicity

Allopurinol decreases the formation of uric acid by inhibiting xanthine oxidase, which catalyses the conversion of hypoxanthine to xanthine and of xanthine to uric acid. Long-term use may lead to xanthine deposits forming in the kidneys.

Kinetics and metabolism

Allopurinol is rapidly absorbed from the gastrointestinal tract under normal conditions.

The half-life of allopurinol in Dalmatian dogs is reported to be 2.7 hours. The half-life of the major metabolite, oxipurinol, is unknown.

Clinical effects

Vomiting, diarrhoea and abdominal tenderness would be anticipated following ingestion of large doses. Excitability and polydipsia have been reported in previous VPISLn cases.

Treatment

Gastric emptying is unlikely to be necessary unless huge quantities (>1 g/kg body weight) have been ingested and the animal presented to surgery within 1 hour. Use of adsorbents is not indicated.

Management is symptomatic and supportive. If there is severe or persistent vomiting, use of metoclopramide may be considered.

Dose: 0.5–1 mg/kg body weight orally, s.c. or i.m. every 6–8 hours; 1–2 mg/kg body weight per day by slow i.v. infusion.

Intravenous fluids may be considered to ensure that the animal remains well hydrated.

References

VPIS (London) past cases up to 97/55047.

Ling GV *et al.* (1997). Pharmacokinetics of allopurinol in Dalmatian dogs. *Journal of Veterinary Pharmacology and Therapeutics* **20(2)**, 134–138.

Alphachloralose

Type of product

Alphachloralose is used as a rodenticide (particularly for mice) and for the control of pest birds (they are immobilised and rendered easier to kill by other means, or die from hypothermia and/or inanition).

Presentation

Commercial and professional products are available in a variety of forms. Some are presented as impregnated wheat or bran granules with an alphachloralose concentration between 2% and 4% w/w. These are often available in small sachets for easy use. One 5 g sachet of a 4% w/w strength will provide 200 mg of alphachloralose.

Professional products may be available in larger containers and at higher concentrations. Some manufacturers colour their products green for identification purposes.

Occurrence of poisoning incidences

Since 1992 the VPIS has handled an average of 20 enquiries per annum concerning accidental ingestion of alphachloralose. Over 85% of these cases involve dogs. Some have developed neurological clinical effects, but all have recovered with symptomatic and supportive treatment.

Toxicity

According to the literature:

- Dogs have been reported to survive doses of 610 mg/kg body weight.
- 660 mg/kg body weight or more may cause fatality.
- The LD_{50} for dogs are quoted in the range 100–600 mg/kg body weight.

In the experience of the VPISLn:

- Ingestion of 73 mg/kg body weight in a cross-bred puppy resulted in weakness, tremors, hyperaesthesia and sedation. The animal recovered with supportive care (VPISLn case 93/48161).
- 208 mg/kg body weight ingested by a 6 kg Jack Russell terrier resulted in severe convulsions within 30 minutes of ingestion. The animal required diazepam and then anaesthesia, but recovered within 24 hours (VPISLn case 95/72705).

Mechanism of toxicity

Alphachloralose causes selective depression of neurones in the ascending reticular formation, thereby suppressing the normal arousal response. In low doses alphachloralose causes increased motor activity but higher doses produce a characteristic CNS depression.

Kinetics and metabolism

Alphachloralose appears to be readily and rapidly absorbed and is reported to be metabolised to chloral and then to trichloroethanol and trichloroacetic acid. In the liver, trichloroethanol combines with glucuronic acid to from urochloralic acid, which is pharmacologically inactive and which is excreted in urine.

Clinical effects

Onset of effects is usually within 1–2 hours. Duration of effects is variable, but cases with effects lasting between 24 and 48 hours have been reported.

Ataxia and hyperactivity are common in the early stages of poisoning. There may also be salivation, weakness and drowsiness, and in severe cases, hypothermia, shallow respiration, weak pulse, coma and convulsions. The usual cause of death is respiratory failure.

Poisoned animals appear to lose sensitivity to pain, but become hypersensitive to touch, sound and electrical stimuli. Dogs have been reported not to respond to normal stimuli or familiar surroundings. Some literature reports describe apparent blindness in dogs.

Treatment

Treatment is necessary for 20 mg/kg body weight, which is equivalent to:

1 g bait/kg body weight for a 2% w/w product

0.5 g bait/kg body weight for a 4% w/w product.

If within 2 hours of ingestion, induce vomiting or consider gastric lavage. Oral adsorbents are not useful.

Emetics:

(a) Apomorphine	Dose:	0.05 mg/kg body weight i.v. or i.m.; 0.1 mg/kg body weight s.c.
(b) Xylazine	Dose:	0.2 mg/kg body weight i.v.; 0.5–1 mg/kg body weight i.m. or s.c.
(c) Ipecacuanha	Dose:	1–2 ml/kg body weight (maximum 20 ml) orally
(d) Soda crystal.		

Treatment thereafter is supportive. Observation for a minimum of 4 hours is recommended.

Where convulsions or severe tremors or hyperaesthesia are present, diazepam or acepromazine may be given.

Diazepam dose: 0.5 mg/kg body weight i.v. repeated every 10 minutes up to three times if needed.

Acepromazine dose: 1–3 mg/kg body weight orally; 0.03–0.1 mg/kg body weight i.m., or s.c.; 0.03 mg/kg body weight by slow i.v. injection. If these fail, then general anaesthesia may be considered for a short while.

Provision of artificial/supplemental heat may be necessary for hypothermia and in severe cases respiratory support may be required.

References

VPIS (London) past cases up to 97/80130.

Foster D (1995). Poisons – Alphachloralose. *In Practice* **17**(8), 381.

Anticoagulant rodenticides

Type of product

The anticoagulants are usually derivatives of either 4-hydroxycoumarin or indane-1,3-dione and are the active constituents of many pesticides preparations for control of infestations of rats and mice.

They are usually of 'first generation' or 'second generation' types. Compounds classified as second generation have a much longer duration of action.

Substances include:

Brodifacoum	Second generation	Coumarin type
Bromadiolone	Second generation	Coumarin type
Chlorphacinone	Second generation	Indandione type
Coumatetralyl	Second generation	Coumarin type
Difenacoum	Second generation	Coumarin type
Diphacinone	Second generation	Indandione type
Flocoumafen	Second generation	Coumarin type
Warfarin	First generation	Coumarin type.

Presentation

Anticoagulants are formulated as ready-to-use baits of variable concentrations. Impregnated powders, grains, seeds and wheat grains are usually of a strength between 0.005–0.01% w/w (equivalent to 50–100 μg anticoagulant/g preparation (ppm)).

Paste, block, gel and liquid preparations tend to be stronger, with concentrations of 0.01–0.25% w/w (equivalent to 100 μg–2.5 mg anticoagulant/g preparation).

Frequently, the preparations are dyed for identification purposes. Many companies use blue or green colours to denote anticoagulant rodenticides, but this is not universally true. In the UK some are coloured purple or red.

In some, anticoagulants may be combined with calciferol of cholecalciferol (see relevant section).

Occurrence of poisoning incidences

Since the launch of the VPIS in 1992 the London centre has received more enquiries about the anticoagulant rodenticides than any other type of product. 117 enquiries were received in 1992 and 268 in 1997. Calls about these products therefore account for 7.5–9% of the total enquiry number.

Over 85% of all these enquiries involved dogs. Difenacoum and bromadiolone are the agents for which most enquiries are received, but this is probably a reflection of the fact that there are more products containing these active ingredients available on the market. Enquiries about chlorphacinone and coumatetralyl are also frequent.

Toxicity

As most rodent bait formulations contain a very small concentration of active ingredient, they are reputedly not highly toxic following small single dose ingestion. However, second generation baits are 'one-shot' baits, designed to kill rodents after one exposure only, and so substantial ingestions by dogs may result in severe toxicity.

Secondary poisonings (i.e. those resulting from ingestion of poisoned rodents) have been reported, and are more likely from second generation anticoagulant-based baits.

According to the literature:

Brodifacoum

- LD_{50} values for brodifacoum in dogs are quoted in the range 0.25–3.5 mg/kg body weight.
- Assuming fatal dose of 0.25 mg/kg body weight and a bait of 0.005% w/w strength, a fatal dose is calculated as 5 g bait/kg body weight in dogs.

Bromadiolone

- LD_{50} values in dogs are quoted in the range 6.3–15 mg/kg body weight.
- Assuming a fatal dose of 6.3 mg/kg body weight and a bait of 0.005% w/w strength, a fatal dose is calculated as 126 g bait/kg body weight.
- Dogs can tolerate repeat doses of 0.5–1.0 mg/kg of bromadiolone for several days.
- Lowest fatal dose reported for bromadiolone is 10 mg/kg.

Chlorphacinone

- LD_{50} values in dogs are quoted in the range 50–100 mg/kg body weight.
- Assuming a fatal dose of 50 mg/kg body weight and a bait of 0.005% w/w strength, a fatal dose of 1 kg bait/kg body weight.

Coumatetralyl

- LD_{50} value in dogs is quoted as 35 mg/kg body weight.
- Assuming a fatal dose of 35 mg/kg body weight and a bait of 0.005% w/w strength, the fatal dose equivalent in dogs is 700 g bait/kg body weight.

Difenacoum

- LD_{50} value for difenacoum in dogs is 50 mg/kg body weight.
- Assuming a fatal dose of 50 mg/kg body weight for difenacoum and a bait of 0.005% w/w strength, a fatal dose in a dog could be as little as 1 kg bait/kg body weight.

Diphacinone

- LD_{50} values in dogs are quoted in the range 1–7.5 mg/kg body weight.
- Assuming a fatal dose of 1 mg/kg body weight and a bait of 0.005% w/w strength, a fatal dose can be calculated as 20 g bait/kg body weight.

Flocoumafen

- LD_{50} value for dogs quoted as 75 μg/kg body weight.
- Assuming a fatal dose of 75 μg/kg body weight and a bait of 0.005% w/w strength, a fatal dose of 1.5 g bait/kg body weight can be calculated.

Warfarin

- LD_{50} values in dogs are quoted in the range 50–300 mg/kg body weight.
- Assuming a fatal dose of 50 mg/kg body weight and a bait of 0.005% strength, then a fatal dose of 1 kg bait/body weight can be calculated.
- Lowest fatal dose is reportedly in the range 20–50 mg/kg body weight.

In the experience of VPISLn:

Brodifacoum

- An 8-year-old Retriever admitted with lethargy, coughing, clotting deficiency, abdominal bleeding was managed with vitamin K_1, antibiotics, plasma expanders and blood transfusion. The animal was found to have liver failure and was euthanased (VPISLn case 94/28809).
- A Jack Russell terrier was admitted with severe vomiting, bruising and renal failure. Vitamin K_1, fluid therapy and peritoneal lavage were given, but the animal died (VPISLn case 96/39725).

Bromadiolone

- A 12-year-old female Border Collie was admitted with posterior paresis, fatigue, tachypnoea, tachycardia, anaemia, intra-abdominal, intestinal, retinal and subcutaneous haemorrhage. She received vitamin K_1 therapy, i.v. fluids, diuretics and, two blood transfusions, but died after 7 days (VPISLn case 91/93238).
- One case of a pregnant bitch presented having eaten a large bag of bromadiolone-based rodenticide. Vitamin K_1 therapy was instituted and the animal delivered a healthy and apparently unaffected litter (VPISLn case 97/41330).

Chlorphacinone

- In general, many more cases presented to veterinarians showing clinical effects.
- Nine fatal cases reported.
- A 15 kg Cocker Spaniel presented with pallor, abdominal tenderness and pulmonary haemorrhage. Condition of animal had deteriorated over 3 weeks. Despite vitamin K_1 and blood transfusions the animal died (VPISLn case 92/23941)
- A 10 kg Terrier cross-bred presented with pale mucous membranes, hyperpnoea and collapse. The dog was given i.v. fluids and vitamin K_1. The animal died (VPISLn case 96/12263).
- A 40 kg Retriever presented 9 days after ingestion of chlorphacinone-containing bait. It was dull and lethargic, hyperpnoeic and tachycardic, had a weak pulse. It was given i.v. fluids, antibiotics, analgesics and died as Vitamin K_1 was being administered (VPISLn case 96/43122).

Coumatetralyl

- No canine fatal cases reported.
- All cases with clinical effects responded well to standard therapies of i.v. fluids, prolonged vitamin K_1 administration, and in some cases blood transfusion.

Difenacoum

- This is the anticoagulant about which VPISLn receives most enquiries.
- Many cases with clinical effects responded well to standard therapies of i.v. fluids, prolonged vitamin K_1 administration, and in some cases blood transfusion.
- A 22 kg cross-bred dog was presented with pale mucous membranes, and elevated PT, and evidence of thoracic haemorrhage. There was significant bleeding from site of venepuncture for collection of sample for PT measurement. The animal received blood transfusion, and prolonged vitamin K_1 and made a full recovery over 4 weeks (VPISLn case 94/16088).
- Several cases have involved animals who were fitting. In these cases, the preparations ingested all contained calciferol as a co-ingredient.

Diphacinone

- A 5 kg Jack Russell terrier presented having collapsed. It had pale mucous membranes, dyspnoea and tachypnoea. Despite prompt vitamin K_1 administration the animal died (VPISLn case 96/61359).

Flocoumafen

- Few cases reported.

- All cases were asymptomatic. Some received emetics and prophylactic vitamin K_1.

Warfarin

- Onset of clinical effects in cases is more rapid, as expected.
- No fatal cases reported to VPISLn.
- All cases with clinical effects responded well to standard therapy of i.v. fluids and prolonged vitamin K_1 administration.

Mechanism of toxicity

Anticoagulants are absorbed from the gastrointestinal tract and act by inhibiting hepatic vitamin K_1 epoxide-reductase, the enzyme responsible for conversion of vitamin K epoxide to vitamin K. This results in the gradual depletion of the body stores of vitamin K needed to convert precursor coagulation proteins to their activated forms. Hence there is a reduction in Factors II (Prothrombin), VII, IX and X and therefore inhibition of prothrombin synthesis within the liver. The anticoagulants achieve this enzyme inhibition by binding reversibly with the proenzyme to form an inactive anticoagulant-coenzyme and displacing vitamin K. Since the reaction is essentially an equilibrium one, administration of vitamin K_1 as therapy will result in increased levels of the vitamin K pro-enzyme (active), hence increasing rate of prothrombin generation and therefore clotting.

The delay to onset of the clinical effects is due to the fact that there is a supply of circulating prothrombin and other vitamin K-dependent clotting factors, which would have to be depleted before clinical effects manifest themselves.

Kinetics and metabolism

Warfarin and the second generation anticoagulants have a relatively slow absorption from the gastrointestinal tract. Over 95% of an ingested warfarin dose is absorbed and approximately 90% absorption occurs for the second generation type.

Warfarin has a plasma half-life in dogs of approximately 14.5 hours. That of the second generation anticoagulants is variable and longer, as they bind strongly to plasma proteins. For example, the plasma half-life of diphacinone is 4–5 days and that of bromadiolone and brodifacoum 6 days. Some have a very long duration of action, however. It is not uncommon for residual effects to be evident some 15–20 days or more post-ingestion, even with antidotal treatment.

Anticoagulants are slowly metabolised by microsomal mixed function oxidases to form inactive metabolites, which are excreted in the urine.

Clinical effects

Clinical effects may be delayed for up to 1–5 days, though are usually seen within 1–3 days of exposure. Duration of effects may be as long as 12–15 days.

Clinical effects include persistent bleeding from the nose, gums, bowel and any wounds, although external bleeding is not always present. Pale mucous membranes, depression, lethargy, weakness, inappetence, anorexia and anaemia are frequent signs. Abdominal tenderness, haematemesis, haematuria and melena are occasionally reported in severe intoxications and are indicative of gastrointestinal haemorrhage. Rarely, respiratory distress (inspiratory and expiratory wheezing) and tachycardia may be noted.

Lameness may occur as a result of swelling around the joints. Pulmonary haemorrhage is indicated by coughing, dyspnoea with moist rales and blood-tinged froth around the nose or mouth.

Sites of venepuncture may bleed excessively.

Haemorrhage into the peritoneal and/or pleural cavities, mediastinum and the cerebral vasculature may occur and subcutaneous swellings, petechial and ecchymotic haemorrhages of the sclera, conjunctiva, and mucous membranes may be seen.

Haemorrhage into vital areas can precipitate rapid fatality (commonly if bleed is into pleural cavity, lung parenchyma, or the pericardial space).

Hypovolaemic shock may occur after rapid blood loss. If the loss is severe, paresis, ataxia, collapse, convulsions and death may occur. Hepatic failure necessitating euthanasia following a serious brodifacoum ingestion, after apparently successful initial management that included blood transfusion, has been reported in VPISLn case 94/28809.

Post-mortem findings

Generalised haemorrhages into body cavities (gastrointestinal lumen, subcutaneous tissues, peritoneum, thorax, lungs, bladder, periarticular areas) are characteristic post-mortem findings. A flaccid rounded heart with sub-epicardial and sub-endocardial haemorrhages may be seen. Severe cases show centrilobular necrosis where hypoxia and anaemia exists.

Laboratory assay of clotting factors or for anticoagulant in biological specimens (ideally liver sample, unclotted blood, stomach and intestinal contents, faeces, spleen and kidney) may help in confirming diagnosis but delay between consumption and the manifestation of effects compounded by metabolism of the anticoagulant may render the anticoagulant hard to detect.

Treatment

Animals with severe coagulopathy require handling with great care to avoid unnecessary stress and risk of haemorrhage, and may require sedation when undergoing treatment.

Treatment is required for any definite or suspected ingestion of more than the following doses or equivalent of the various anticoagulants by a dog:

Brodifacoum	3 g/kg body weight of a 0.005% w/w bait
Bromadiolone	100 g/kg body weight of a 0.005% w/w bait
Chlorphacinone	750 g/kg body weight of a 0.005% w/w bait
Coumatetralyl	500 g/kg body weight of a 0.005% w/w bait
Difenacoum	750 g/kg body weight of a 0.005% w/w bait
Diphacinone	15 g/kg body weight of a 0.005% w/w bait
Flocoumafen	1 g/kg body weight of a 0.005% w/w bait
Warfarin	750 g/kg body weight of a 0.005% w/w bait.

Simple blood tests can confirm diagnosis – clotting or prothrombin time (PT) would both be significantly elevated. PT is the most useful indicator as it measures clotting factor VII, which has the shortest half-life of the affected clotting factors. Care must also be taken when taking samples for PT determination, as the site of venepuncture may bleed excessively. The smallest possible needle should be used.

Ideally, samples should be taken prior to antidotal therapy with vitamin K_1.

If the animal is presented within 2 hours of the ingestion, induce emesis, if this can be achieved safely. Ideally, follow this with adsorbent administration.

Emetics:

(a) Apomorphine	Dose:	0.05 mg/k body weight i.v. or i.m.; 0.1 mg/kg body weight s.c.
(b) Xylazine	Dose:	0.2 mg/kg body weight i.v.; 0.5–1 mg/kg body weight i.m. or s.c.
(c) Ipecacuanha	Dose:	1–2 ml/kg body weight (maximum 20 ml) orally
(d) Soda crystal.		

Adsorbents:

(a) Activated charcoal	Dose:	2 g/kg body weight orally
(b) BCK granules®	Dose:	6–18 g orally 2–3 times daily.

If the animal is symptomatic, then a blood sample for determination of PT should be taken and then vitamin K_1 administered. Dose: 2–5 mg/kg body weight *i.m.* or *s.c.* at multiple injection sites.

Notes

1. Intravenous administration of vitamin K_1 is best avoided unless ingestion was very recent, as the site of venepuncture may bleed excessively. For all parenteral administrations, the smallest possible needle should be used.

2. Some vitamin K_1 preparations are reported to induce anaphylactic reactions upon intravenous administration. Care should be taken to check instructions for vitamin K_1 preparation used.

3. Synthetic vitamin K compounds that require metabolic modification before they are active should not be given.

4. Pregnancy is no contra-indication to vitamin K_1 therapy. In one literature report (Hornfeldt and Phearman, 1996) and one VPISLn case (97/41330) it has been given to pregnant bitches with potential poisoning with no adverse outcome.

5. Vitamin K_1 is phytomenadione.

Vitamin K_1 administration should start to reverse any hypoprothrombinaemia within an hour or so, with a full effect being noticeable at about 4–6 hours. If possible check PT at least 4–6 hours after the initial vitamin K_1 dosing.

In ALL cases the PT should be measured on a daily basis for a minimum of 3 days.

In asymptomatic animals, if the PT remains normal for 3 days after exposure, then further treatment is unlikely to be required.

If the PT is elevated, then parenteral vitamin K_1 administration should be started or continued on a daily basis at a dosage of 2–5 mg/kg body weight *i.m.* or *s.c.* at multiple injection sites until PT normalises.

Once PT has normalised, the animal should continue to receive vitamin K_1 orally for 2–3 weeks at an initial dosage of 2–5 mg/kg body weight in divided doses, gradually reducing the dose over this period (recommended reduction of 50% per week). Ideally, some reassessment of the coagulation status should be made after 2–3 weeks and before the treatment is discontinued and also 3 days after treatment has ceased to ensure no relapse occurs.

Severe intoxications:

If the animal has severe anaemia associated with dyspnoea but without pulmonary or thoracic bleeding, then whole blood transfusions may be necessary to increase blood volume and levels of clotting factors.

Regimen recommended is 20 ml/kg body weight – administer half this dose rapidly and the remainder by slow i.v. drip. The whole blood must be fresh, as factors V and VIII are labile on storage.

If dyspnoea is related to haemorrhage within the pulmonary or thoracic area, then bleeding sites need to be identified and thoracentesis considered.

Hypovolaemic shock requires fluid replacement and may also require blood transfusion, and maintenance of renal output.

Supplemental iron and vitamins, particularly Vitamin B_{12}, may be needed.

References and further reading

VPIS (London) past cases up to 97/156004.

Clark AM (1981). Rat bait poisoning. *Veterinary Record* **109(18)**, 413.

Cranna GR (1987). Toxicity associated with insecticides – a perspective. In *Veterinary Clinical Toxicology, Proceedings No. 103* (Proceedings of a conference held at the University of Sydney, Australia, 24–28 August 1987), pp. 63–83.

Dorman DC (1990). Anticoagulant, cholecalciferol and bromethalin-based rodenticides. *Veterinary Clinics of North America: Small Animal Practice* **20(2)**, 339–352.

DuVall MD *et al.* (1989). Case studies on second generation anticoagulant rodenticide toxicities in non-target species. *Journal of Veterinary Diagnostic Investigation* **1**, 66–68.

Hornfeldt CS and Phearman S (1996). Successful treatment of brodifacoum poisoning in a pregnant bitch. *Journal of the American Veterinary Medical Association* **209(10)**, 1690–1691.

Kammermann-Luescher B (1978). Cumarinvergiftung bei Hund und Katze. *Schweizer Archiv für Tierheilkunde* **120**, 231–244.

Lewis DC *et al.* (1997). Thrombocytopaenia in dogs with anticoagulant rodenticide-induced hemorrhage: eight cases (1990–1995). *Journal of the American Animal Hospital Association* **33**, 417–422.

McSporran KD and Phillips CA (1983). Brodifacoum poisoning in a dog. *New Zealand Veterinary Journal* **31**, 185–186.

Maver S (1990). Poison – coumarin derivatives. *In Practice* **12(4)**, 174–175.

Mount ME (1988). Diagnosis and therapy of anticoagulant rodenticide intoxications *Veterinary Clinics of North America: Small Animal Practice* **18(1)**, 115–130.

Mount ME and Feldman BF (1983). Mechanism of diphacinone rodenticide toxicosis in the dog and its therapeutic indications. *American Journal of Veterinary Research* **44(11)**, 2009–2017.

Neff-Davis CA *et al.* (1981). Warfarin in the dog; pharmacokinetics as related to clinical response. *Journal of Veterinary Pharmacology and Therapeutics* **4**, 135–140.

Oehme FW (1987). Agricultural pesticide toxicity in domestic animals. In *Veterinary Clinical Toxicology, Proceedings No. 103* (Proceedings of a conference at the University of Sydney, Australia, 24–28 August, 1987), pp. 429–440.

Oehme FW (1987). Clinical toxicology in small animals. In *Veterinary Clinical Toxicology, Proceedings No. 103* (Proceedings of a conference at the University of Sydney, Australia, 24–28 August, 1987), pp. 443–476.

Schulman A *et al.* (1986). Diphacinone-induced coagulopathy in the dog. *Journal of the American Veterinary Medical Association* **188(4)**, 402–405.

Stowe CM *et al.* (1983). Apparent brodifacoum poisoning in a dog. *Journal of the American Veterinary Medical Association* **182(8)**, 817–818.

Talcott PA and Dorman DC (1997). Pesticide exposures in companion animals. *Veterinary Medicine* **92(2)**, 167–182.

Veenstra GE *et al.* (1991). Metabolic and toxicological studies on the anticoagulant rodenticide, flocoumafen. *Archives of Toxicology* **14**(suppl.), 160–165.

Woody BJ *et al.* (1992). Coagulopathic effects and therapy of brodifacoum toxicosis in dogs. *Journal of Veterinary Internal Medicine* **6**, 23–28.

Baclofen

Type of product

Baclofen is a skeletal muscle relaxant derived from the inhibitory neurotransmitter gamma-aminobutyric acid (GABA). It is used in human medicine as a treatment for chronic muscle spasm or control of muscle spasticity due to, for example, multiple sclerosis, spinal cord injuries and cerebral palsy.

Presentation

Baclofen is available in the UK in both tablet and liquid forms. Tablets are commonly of 10 mg strength and the liquid of 1 mg/ml. It is a prescription-only medicine.

Occurrence of poisoning incidences

Since the launch of the VPIS in 1992 there has been an average of 10 enquiries per year concerning baclofen ingestion in dogs. There have also been a few isolated feline cases. In all canine cases bar one the animals have shown severe clinical effects, often despite low dosings. Several fatal cases have been documented.

Recommended dosage

In the UK the drug is supplied for use in humans only.

Toxicity

Baclofen toxicity usually causes sudden rapid onset of clinical effects, which are usually severe and may have a duration of well over 48 hours.

In the experience of the VPISLn:

- A dose of 1 mg/kg body weight produced ataxia, profound sedation, salivation, hypothermia and collapse. The animal survived (VPISLn case 87/37030).
- In two cases between 24 and 30 mg/kg body weight of baclofen was ingested by dogs, with fatal results, despite aggressive supportive therapy. Both animals were tachycardic, unresponsive, tachypnoeic, hypersalivating, and eventually collapsed. One dog developed severe fitting (VPISLn cases 93/14178 and 95/31610).
- One dog consumed a potential 80 mg/kg body weight dose of baclofen. Despite drowsiness, bradycardia with subsequent collapse, coma and

severe hypothermia the animal survived with supportive care over a 72 hour period (VPISLn 94/40332).

Mechanism of toxicity

The clinical effects seen in poisoning cases can be attributed to inhibition of CNS reflexes. Its effects are most pronounced in the spinal cord. Baclofen has little activity on $GABA_A$ receptors but binds well to presynaptic $GABA_B$ receptors, thereby reducing transmitter release, perhaps by a reduction in presynaptic calcium ion influx. It has some possible post-synaptic action meditated through increase in potassium ion permeability, with a resulting control of neuronal excitability.

Kinetics and metabolism

Little animal data are available. It would appear that the drug is rapidly absorbed in dogs and that the drug has a long elimination half-life.

Baclofen is excreted in the urine.

Clinical effects

The onset of clinical effects is often very sudden and usually within 1 hour of ingestion. Recovery from clinical effects may take from 36–96 hours.

The most common features reported are early excitability, salivation, constricted or pin-point pupils, weakness, ataxia, twitching, tremor, bradycardia, pale mucous membranes, drowsiness, loss of swallowing reflexes and collapse. In severe cases cyanosis, coma, convulsions, shock, hypothermia, tachycardia and respiratory distress may occur. In many cases reported to the VPIS the animals were vocalising markedly.

Treatment

Treatment is necessary for any amount.

If within 2 hours of ingestion induce vomiting, after ensuring there is an adequate swallowing reflex. Then administer adsorbents.

Where the swallowing reflex is reduced or absent, give adsorbents only.

Emetics:

(a) Apomorphine	Dose:	0.05 mg/kg body weight i.v. or i.m.; 0.1 mg/kg body weight s.c.
(b) Xylazine	Dose:	0.2 mg/kg body weight i.v.; 0.5–1 mg/kg body weight i.m. or s.c.
(c) Ipecacuanha	Dose:	1–2 ml/kg body weight (maximum 20 ml) orally
(d) Soda crystal.		

Adsorbents:

(a) Activated charcoal Dose: 2 g/kg body weight orally
(b) BCK granules® Dose: 6–18 g orally 2–3 times daily.

Treatment thereafter is supportive. Observe for a minimum of 4 hours.

Diazepam or acepromazine may be given for muscle tremor or to control convulsions. Where adsorbents have been administered, then use parenteral routes. Diazepam dose: 0.5 mg/kg body weight i.v. repeated every 10 minutes up to three times if needed; acepromazine dose: 1–3 mg/kg body weight orally; 0.03–0.1 mg/kg body weight i.m., or s.c.; 0.03 mg/kg body weight by slow i.v. injection.

Atropine may be given for severe bradycardia. Atropine dose: 30–100 μg/kg body weight s.c. or i.m.; 20 μg/kg body weight i.v.

Provision of artificial/supplemental heat may be necessary for hypothermia.

Doxapram has been used in a few past VPIS cases as a respiratory stimulant. Dose: 2–10 mg/kg body weight by i.v. injection.

Reference

VPIS (London) past cases up to 97/170000.

Batteries

Presentation

This varies. The types of batteries most commonly implicated in animal poisoning incidences are the miniature cell or button battery or the small AA or AAA devices used for charging calculators, electronic games, watches, hearing aids, photographic equipment, remote controls, portable telephones and pagers.

Most batteries contain either strong acids, e.g. sulphuric acid, or strong alkalis, e.g. potassium hydroxide, as the conducting medium and many have a significant metal content. Some button batteries still contain mercury as mercuric chloride, a soluble salt.

Occurrence of poisoning incidences

Since the launch of the VPIS in 1992 an average of 10 cases per year involving small battery ingestion by dogs have been reported to the London centre. In some cases, the batteries have been swallowed with the machine they supply, e.g. mobile phones. No fatal outcomes have been reported, although some animals have displayed signs consistent with exposure to the corrosive contents of the cells.

Toxicity

Small batteries, if ingested, are capable of producing both corrosive and toxic effects, which may be multifactorial in origin. While the majority of batteries traverse the gastrointestinal tract uneventfully, complications may arise if the battery becomes lodged. In man this occurs most commonly in the oesophagus, but has been reported at other sites.

Mechanisms of toxicity

Damage to the battery casing may occur in the gut, from acidic attack by gastric acid and/or electrolytic attack due to its own electrical properties, causing leakage of the contents. Leakage and/or production (by hydrolysis of water) of corrosive conducting media may cause severe caustic injury, while leakage of metal salts may result in systemic toxicity. A single mercury button battery contains sufficient mercuric chloride to deliver a potential lethal dose for a small dog.

Tissue damage may also occur from prolonged contact at a single site as the electrical activity of the battery causes local short circuit through the tissues, as well as a rise in pH.

Theoretically, used batteries pose less of a hazard since they are less likely to leak or cause electrical damage and in spent mercury batteries the mercuric chloride will be largely reduced to harmless elemental mercury. However, it is important to remember that batteries that do not drive their intended appliances may still retain some residual charge and, in the case of mercury batteries, some unreduced mercuric salt.

Clinical effects

In most symptomatic cases reported to the VPIS (London) the animals show evidence of having bitten through the battery casing and therefore have local irritant and corrosive effects to the mouth and oesophagus.

Oesophageal impaction may result in irritability, difficulty in swallowing, salivation, vomiting and, in theory, local burns. Clinical effects from corrosion or perforation may be delayed.

Batteries which open in the lower gut may cause vomiting, tarry or bloody stools, and abdominal tenderness.

In the case of mercury batteries, signs of mercury intoxication, initially severe gastrointestinal upset, may be delayed by several days.

Treatment

Emesis and gastric lavage are not recommended, since these procedures are unlikely to evacuate batteries owing to their density and the risk that they may lodge in oesophagus. Use of adsorbents is not routinely advocated as they are of limited benefit and will obscure detection of the batteries and discolour the stools.

The brand and type of battery should be determined where possible. Spare batteries may be kept at home and may bear an identifying code that poisons information centres use to identify the type involved.

X-rays should be taken where practicable to confirm ingestion and to determine the position of the battery. The condition of the battery may also be determined as contents are radiopaque.

If the battery is still in the oesophagus prompt removal is advocated, by endoscopy where possible.

When batteries are intact and in the stomach or beyond, laxatives may be given to promote transit through the gastrointestinal tract. Ideally, X-rays should be repeated to monitor the passage of the battery through the gut until passed in the stools. Surgical removal is indicated when there is no movement of the battery in a 48 hour period, the battery shows evidence of leakage, or if there is clinical evidence of significant gastroenteritis or discoloured stools.

References and further reading

VPIS (London) past cases up to 97/115955.

Campbell A, Bates N and Farrow C (1997). Button batteries. In Bates, N, Edwards, N, Roper J and Volans G (eds), *Paediatric Toxicology*. London: Macmillan, pp. 103–108.

Blue–green algae / Cyanobacteria

Description and occurrence

Blue–green algae are primitive plants/organisms with many characteristics of both bacteria and algae. They are capable of photosynthesis, the chlorophyll giving them the observed blue–green colour in many cases, and some are also able to fix gaseous nitrogen.

Blue–green algae are found in fresh, brackish and marine waterbodies throughout the UK. In any location there may be many different types co-existing. The type(s) present in any waterbody depend on many factors, including size of waterbody, light penetration, and nutrient availability. Macroscopically, blue–green algae have a granular appearance but they grow as single cells, cell clusters and filaments, often surrounded by a mucinous sheath. Under favourable conditions, when the weather is sunny, temperature of the water high, and water nutrients, especially nitrogen and phosphorus, are abundant, the blue–green algae may form massive growths or blooms. These are either floating, 'planktonic', or bottom-dwelling or 'benthic'. These blooms occur most commonly in late spring, summer and early autumn.

Normally, blue–green algae can regulate their own buoyancy as they possess intracellular air/gas filled vesicles or vacuoles by which they control their density, thereby remaining in the area of optimum growth conditions. Under rapidly changing conditions, for example if strong wind conditions are present or if water is disturbed, they lose this ability and may float to the top forming scums or sink to the bottom. This may also occur if the cell growth rate becomes too high and cells reaching less favourable water areas die. The scums vary in colour, ranging from green to blue–green but also from red to brown or black.

Under less optimal conditions of light, nutrients or temperature, the cells die or deteriorate and release their toxins. Often winds blow the algal scums that form on waterbody surfaces to the shore, concentrating them and making them more accessible to the animals who may be at risk from exposure.

Genera include:

Microcystis	freshwater	planktonic
Anabaena	freshwater	planktonic
Aphanizomenon	freshwater	planktonic
Gloeotrichia	freshwater	
Nodularia	freshwater	planktonic
Nostoc	freshwater	planktonic
Oscillatoria	freshwater	planktonic/benthic.

Occurrence of poisoning incidences

Since 1992 the VPIS London centre has received a small number of enquiries every year regarding blue–green algae exposures in animals, predominantly dogs. Although the number of enquiries is small, except in very hot summers, a significant number of reported exposures result in fatalities in the animals concerned.

Toxicity

Many blue–green algae contain or produce a variety of toxins, although not all are toxic. There are more than 40 toxic species documented. Exposures in animals usually occur when they drink water from ponds or waterbodies where the algae have bloomed. In dogs, exposures have occurred as a result of the animals swimming in such locations and also from grooming after skin exposures. The toxins produced by the blue–green algae have a high acute toxicity and exposures frequently result in fatality. Death is usually very rapid. Blue–green algae have also caused fatalities in sheep, cattle, and birds. Animals may occasionally be found dead at the water's edge.

It is calculated that concentrated scums at waterbody shores or edges present a toxic or lethal dose of blue–green algal toxins in fluid volumes far less than the daily fluid requirement of the animals who may drink the water there.

Mechanism of toxicity

The mechanisms of toxicity of the various blue–green algae are dependent on the species to which the animal has becomes exposed, as well as that of the animal that has been exposed. Toxicity is also dependent on dose ingested, as well as the stage of decomposition of the algae.

Some species contain or produce hepatotoxins. These are usually cyclic peptides, which cause dysfunctional phosphorylation of cellular keratins, thereby disrupting normal cytoskeletal structure. This leads to rounding of the hepatocytes, disruption of the hepatic sinusoidal epithelium, hepato-cyte separation and hepatic necrosis and failure. Hepatic haemorrhage may also occur. Depletion of coagulation factors and also nephritis have been reported following exposures to blue–green algae of the hepatotoxic variety. Fatalities resulting from exposure to this type of algae normally occur as a result of hepatic necrosis, haemorrhage and hypovolaemic shock. Some of the hepatotoxins are potent tumour promoters as well, which may have implications for animals that survive the exposure.

The hepatotoxins produced by species from the *Microcystis* genera have been well studied and characterised. They are cyclic heptapeptides and are named microcystins. These are released on cell death. Those produced by species of *Nodularia* are cyclic pentapeptides called nodularins.

Other blue–green algae contain or produce neurotoxins. Some of these have been isolated and characterised. *Anabaena* and *Oscillatoria* species both produce a bicyclic secondary amine alkaloid called anatoxin-*a* (previously called VFDF, very fast death factor), which is a depolarising agent. It is a structural analogue of cocaine. It acts at nicotinic receptors causing respiratory paralysis. These species, together with those of the *Aphanizomenon* genera may also produce an unstable cholinesterase inhibitor, with an organophosphate structure, named anatoxin-a(s). This produces salivation and increase in mucous secretions, tremors, convulsions, ataxia, cyanosis and respiratory failure. The *Aphanizomenon* genera also produce two similar neurotoxins called saxitoxin and neosaxitoxin, as well as three related compounds of similar structure. Saxitoxin and neosaxitoxin are fast-acting sodium channel blockers. Saxitoxin is the agent of paralytic shellfish poisoning.

Additionally, the cell walls of many of the blue–green algae species contain lipopolysaccharide endotoxins. These are irritant to mucous membranes and skin. It is thought that some of the gastrointestinal clinical effects may be in part due to the irritant nature of these endotoxins.

Clinical effects

Onset of clinical effects may be within 15 minutes of exposure, and usually occurs within 1 hour. Deaths may occur rapidly, often within 10–30 minutes of the onset of clinical effects and usually within 24 hours of the original exposure.

Gastrointestinal upset is often the primary presenting sign whatever species of blue–green algae are involved, and often preludes development of more severe effects. The common gastrointestinal features are acute vomiting, haematemesis, abdominal tenderness and, more rarely, diarrhoea, which may be haemorrhagic.

The other clinical effects are wide-ranging as they depend on the type(s) of toxins involved, since many exposures are to several different types simultaneously.

Common features observed include salivation, pale mucous membranes, piloerection, lethargy, generalised weakness, incoordination, ataxia, collapse, hyperaesthesia, muscle fasciculation, tremors, convulsions, bradycardia, dyspnoea, tachypnoea, cyanosis and coma. Often development is so rapid that respiratory distress, collapse, convulsions and death may be seen within 15 minutes of exposure.

Dogs that have been exposed to blue–green algae of the hepatotoxic variety may exhibit clinical effects over a longer time period. There may be evidence of haemorrhage, hypotension or hypovolaemic shock and icterus. Liver failure and also nephritis may develop. There may be elevated liver enzymes (ALT, Gamma GT, aspartate aminotransferase, alkaline phosphatase), elevated bile acids and evidence of renal impairment (elevated creatinine and urea). Some animals have developed photosensitisation.

Post-mortem findings

These vary dependent on the type of algae to which the animal was exposed.

Those exposed to the neurotoxin-producing variety who succumb rapidly may not display gross lesions. There is frequently lung congestion, cyanosed mucous membranes and central nervous system congestion. Cyanobacteria may be isolated in stomach contents.

Those exposed to the hepatotoxic blue–green algae may have an enlarged and haemorrhagic liver, fluid or blood-filled body cavities, petechial haemorrhage and ecchymoses. Microscopic analysis may reveal rounded and dissociated hepatocytes and centrilobular to hepatic necrosis. Cyanobacteria may also be isolated in stomach and intestinal contents.

Treatment

Speed is essential.

The animal should be removed from the source of exposure and either given a gastric lavage or emesis should be induced. Adsorbents should be given if practicable.

Emetics:

(a) Apomorphine	Dose:	0.05 mg/kg body weight i.v. or i.m.; 0.1 mg/kg body weight s.c.
(b) Xylazine	Dose:	0.2 mg/kg body weight i.v.; 0.5–1 mg/kg body weight i.m. or s.c.
(c) Ipecacuanha	Dose:	1–2 ml/kg body weight (maximum 20 ml) orally
(d) Soda crystal.		

Adsorbents:

(a) Activated charcoal	Dose:	2 g/kg body weight orally
(b) BCK granules®	Dose:	6–18 g orally 2–3 times daily.

Once the animal has been stabilised, the coat should be thoroughly washed and the animal collared to prevent grooming.

Management is thereafter largely supportive. The dogs should be kept adequately hydrated and electrolytes checked and corrected if symptomatic. In some cases, antibiotics have been administered and glucose, calcium and magnesium supplementation instituted. The animals should be kept out of direct sunlight.

Diazepam should be given if there is severe muscle twitching or convulsant activity. Diazepam dose: 0.5 mg/kg body weight i.v. repeated every 10 minutes up to three times if needed.

If the animal is exhibiting cholinergic signs, then use of atropine may be considered. In theory, since the neurotoxin causing these signs is an organophosphate derivative, use of pralidoxime, which is an antidotal therapy for organophosphate poisoning, may be considered as an adjunct to atropine therapy.

Atropine dose: 0.2–2 mg/kg body weight to effect (one-quarter of dose given i.v. and the remainder i.m. or s.c.). The dose may be repeated as required (usually every 45–90 minutes initially). Large doses may be required.

Pralidoxime dose: 20–50 mg/kg body weight by slow i.v. injection (over 2 minutes at least and at a dose no more than 500 mg/minute) or i.m. or s.c. Recovery will not be immediate but over a 24–48 hour period.

In general, use of morphine, succinylcholine, barbiturates and phenothiazines should be avoided because their effects will be enhanced by organophosphate presence.

Investigative

Where possible, monitor liver and kidney function by measurement of liver enzymes and urea and creatinine. If there is evidence of haemorrhage, then clotting profile should be checked.

Cyanobacteria may be identified in scums from coats or in vomitus. This may be useful in confirming exposure.

References and further reading

VPIS (London) past cases up to 97/104889.

National Rivers Authority (1990). *Toxic blue-green algae*, Water quality series, Vol. 2. London: National Rivers Authority.

Beasley VR *et al*. 1989. Diagnostic and clinically important aspects of cyanobacterial (blue-green algae) toxicoses. *Journal of Veterinary Diagnostic Investigation* **1**, 359–365.

Codd GA *et al*. (1992). Fatal attraction to cyanobacteria? *Nature* **359**, 110–111.

Corkhill N *et al*. (1989). Poisoning at Rutland Water. *Veterinary Record* **125(13)**, 356.

Edney ATB (1990). Algal poisoning. *Veterinary Record* **126(12)**, 297–298.

Edwards C *et al*. (1992). Identification of anatoxin-*a* in benthic cyanobacteria (blue-green algae) and in associated dog poisonings at Loch Insh, Scotland. *Toxicon* **30(10)**, 1165–1175.

Elder GH *et al*. (1993). Hazardous freshwater cyanobacteria (blue-green algae). *The Lancet* **341**, 1519–1520.

Gunn GJ (1992). Poison – cyanobacteria (blue-green algae). *In Practice* **14(3)**, 132–133.

Gunn GJ *et al*. (1991). Additional algal toxicosis hazard. *Veterinary Record* **129(17)**, 391.

Gunn GJ *et al*. (1992). Fatal canine neurotoxicosis attributed to blue-green algae. *Veterinary Record* **130(14)**, 301–302.

Harding WR *et al*. (1995). Death of a dog attributed to the cyanobacterial (blue-green algal) hepatoxtoxin nodularin in South Africa. *Journal of the South African Veterinary Association* **66(4)**, 256–259.

Henriksen P *et al.* (1997). Detection of an anatoxin-a(s)-like anticholinesterase in natural blooms and cultures of cyanobacteria/blue-green algae from Danish lakes and in the stomach contents of poisoned birds. *Toxicon* **35(6)**, 901–913.

Mahmood NA *et al.* (1988). Anticholinesterase poisonings in dogs from a cyanobacterial (blue-green algae) bloom dominated by *Anabaena flos-aquea*. *American Journal of Veterinary Research* **49(4)**, 500–503.

Tyagi MB *et al.* (1999). Cyanobacterial toxins: the current status. *Journal of Microbiology and Biotechnology* **9(1)**, 9–21.

Borax

Type of product

Borax (sodium borate) is a constituent of many liquid ant or cockroach killer preparations. Borates have some use in mouthwashes, contact lens solutions, liquid medical preparations such as eye drops, and some soaps and detergents.

Presentation

Liquid ant or roach killers are usually sugary solutions containing borax at a concentration of 5–7%. The sugary nature of the liquids makes the insecticides palatable and attractive to pets.

Occurrence of poisoning incidences

Since the launch of the VPIS in 1992 the London centre has received between 20 and 30 enquiries a year concerning borax insecticide ingestion by dogs. Less than 20% of the animals involved developed any clinical effects.

Toxicity

The toxicity of borax is unclear. Ingestion of borax insecticides rarely results in more than mild gastrointestinal effects. Few fatal cases are documented, and those that are provide limited data.

According to the literature:

- Lowest published lethal dose for dogs is 3 g/kg body weight.
- Other papers report no clinical effects other than vomiting at doses from 1.54–6.51 g/kg body weight.

Mechanism of toxicity

The mechanism of toxicity is unknown, but concentrated borax solutions are irritant to skin and mucous membranes.

Kinetics and metabolism

Borax is readily absorbed from the gastrointestinal tract and across mucous membranes and abraded skin. It is concentrated in kidneys and slowly excreted unchanged in urine. Approximately 40–60% will be excreted within 12–24 hours of exposure.

Clinical effects

Serious cases are rare. Clinical effects usually have an onset of about 2 hours at most.

Commonly occurring signs are those of buccal and gastrointestinal irritation, particularly vomiting, diarrhoea, abdominal tenderness and salivation. Shivering, shaking, tremors, ataxia, drowsiness and depression have been reported in several VPISLn cases. In a few cases pyrexia, polydipsia, fitting and collapse have been reported. Skin exposures may result in erythema.

In the literature, the following effects have been reported in small animal exposures: generalised muscle weakness, coma, Cheyne-Stokes respiration, convulsions, acidosis and electrolyte imbalances, disseminated intravascular coagulation, shock, and renal impairment characterised by oliguria or anuria.

Post-mortem findings

Few data are available, but in theory congestion of gastrointestinal tract, kidneys and liver would be anticipated. There may be evidence of cerebral oedema.

Treatment

Emesis is probably not necessary following ingestion of ant or cockroach killer liquids containing borax at concentrations up to 10% in strength. Following ingestion of more concentrated products, emesis should be induced if the animal presents to surgery within 2 hours.

Emetics:

(a) Apomorphine   Dose: 0.05 mg/kg body weight i.v. or i.m.; 0.1 mg/kg body weight s.c.

(b) Xylazine   Dose: 0.2 mg/kg body weight i.v.; 0.5–1 mg/kg body weight i.m. or s.c.

(c) Ipecacuanha   Dose: 1–2 ml/kg body weight (maximum 20 ml) orally

(d) Soda crystal.

Borates and borax bind poorly to activated charcoal and therefore the use of adsorbents is not advocated.

Treatment thereafter is supportive with fluid replacement, washing of exposed skin where appropriate, and use of anticonvulsants such as diazepam if necessary.

Diazepam dose: 0.5 mg/kg body weight i.v. repeated every 10 minutes up to three times if needed.

In severe cases, if the animal is oliguric or anuric, renal function should be monitored.

Investigative

In cases where severe clinical effects are observed then electrolytes, blood gasses and renal function should be monitored.

Boric acid can be detected in urine and blood, which could be used to confirm a diagnosis of borax ingestion.

A boron blood level above 50 μg/ml would be considered toxic.

References and further reading

VPIS (London) past cases up to 97/57816.

Coppock RW et al. (1988). The toxicity of detergents, bleaches, antiseptics and disinfectants in small animals. Veterinary and Human Toxicology 30(5), 463–473.

Kiesche-Nesselrodt A and Hooser SB (1990). Boric acid. Veterinary Clinics of North America: Small Animal Practice 20(2), 369–373.

Talcott PA and Dorman DC (1997). Pesticide exposures in companion animals. Veterinary Medicine 92(2), 167–181.

Calciferol / Vitamin D₂ and Cholecalciferol / Vitamin D₃

Type of product

Calciferol (vitamin D_2) is found in vitamin preparations, cod liver oil, in some veterinary preparations – especially injections used to prevent parturient paresis (hypocalcaemia after birth). It has occasionally been used as a growth promoter in dogs. Most importantly, it has a use as a rodenticide either on its own or in combination with second generation anticoagulant compounds such as brodifacoum, bromadiolone and difenacoum (see anticoagulant rodenticide entry). The rodenticides produce delayed toxicosis – they are designed to cause death in rodents 1–3 days after a single ingestion.

Cholecalciferol (vitamin D_3) is the glycoside of 1,25-dihydroxycholecalciferol, the metabolite of calciferol. It is found naturally in the plants *Solanum malacoxylon*, *Trisetum flavescens* and *Cestrum diurnum*. Cholecalciferol also has use in rodenticide preparations.

Both calciferol and cholecalciferol may also be found in feed additives.

Presentation

Calciferol exists in its natural state as colourless prismatic crystals; cholecalciferol as fine needle-shaped crystals. Both are insoluble in water and soluble in most organic solvents. Both are slightly soluble in vegetable oils.

In rodenticide preparations the strengths usually range between 0.1% w/w in combination preparations to about 4% w/w in preparations with calciferol or cholecalciferol alone. These presentations vary considerably in appearance. They may be liquids for mixture with grain or biscuit, or exist in seed or grain impregnated with the compound prior to sale.

Occurrence of poisoning incidences

Since the launch of the VPIS in 1992 enquiries about rodenticides containing calciferol or cholecalciferol as an ingredient have risen from six in 1992 to 17 in 1997, representing about 0.6% of the annual enquiries on average. All these enquiries have involved dogs.

Enquiries about vitamin D as a drug or part of a multivitamin combination have remained more or less constant, with less than 10 enquiries handled per year.

Only the anticoagulant combination preparations have resulted in clinical effects.

Toxicity

When the calciferol and cholecalciferol rodenticides were introduced, it was claimed that they were less toxic to non-target species than some of the other rodenticides available. Subsequent clinical experience has shown that these compounds pose a significant threat for both dogs and cats.

Excessive use of growth promoters in large-breed dogs has led to toxicosis. In overdose or following accidental ingestion and absorption, hypercalcaemia may result. This may cause cardiac conduction defects or cardiac failure. Also soft tissue receptors respond to one of the metabolites, 1,25-Dihydroxycholecalciferol (1,25-dihydroxyvitamin D), resulting in abnormal tissue mineralisation. Critical tissues affected are the renal tubules and small to medium arterioles.

High concentrations of active cholecalciferol/vitamin D$_3$ may cause direct cellular degeneration and necrosis.

According to the literature:

- The acute oral LD$_{50}$ in dogs for calciferol is quoted as 85 mg/kg body weight.
- The acute oral LD$_{50}$ in dogs for cholecalciferol is quoted as 88 mg/kg body weight.
- Clinical reports indicate toxicosis at ingested doses of 0.5–5 mg/kg body weight.
- Fatal intoxications are reported at doses of 10–20 mg/kg body weight.
- The lowest published lethal dose for calciferol ingestion in dogs is 4 mg/kg body weight.
- Fatalities in dogs for cholecalciferol ingestions of 2–3 mg/kg body weight are documented.

Gradual accumulation from prolonged exposure to lower doses may lead to toxicity.

Dogs with pre-existing kidney disease are predisposed to calciferol/cholecalciferol toxicosis.

Conversions

Vitamin D 1 mg = 41 000 IU approx.

Mechanism of toxicity

Calciferol and cholecalciferol are rapidly absorbed and metabolised. The parent compounds and the intermediate metabolites have some limited pharmacological action but the major toxic effects are due to the major metabolite, calcitriol, which enhances resorption of calcium from bone, absorption of calcium from the gut, intestinal calcium transport and proximal renal tubule resorption of calcium in the kidney. This gives rise to hypercalcaemia and toxicity.

Kinetics and metabolism

Absorption of calciferol/cholecalciferol is rapid and complete in the small intestine. A high lipid diet will increase absorption. It is carried in plasma to the liver and kidneys. It is metabolised in the liver to 25-hydroxycholecalciferol (25-hydroxyvitamin D), which is converted to the physiologically active 1,25-dihydroxycholecalciferol (1,25-dihydroxyvitamin D), otherwise called calcitriol, in the kidney.

Calciferol/cholecalciferol metabolites are excreted primarily via bile and in the faeces. Less than one-third is excreted in the urine.

Serum half-life of 25-hydroxycholecalciferol (25-hydroxyvitamin D) is quoted as 10.67 days.

Case report

VPISLn case report 94/28405.

A dog was re-presented to surgery some 4 days after ingesting a rodenticide assumed to be of an anticoagulant type, having been on Vitamin K$_1$ since its initial presentation on day 1. The dog displayed marked polydipsia in the absence of any other clinical effects. Management was supportive. On day 7 it was found to have hypercalcaemia of 4.02 mmol/L (equivalent to 16.3 mg/dl). The normal upper limit is usually quoted as 3 mmol/L (approximately equivalent to 12.1 mg/dl). This biochemical finding combined with an altered history from the dog's owner, led to a diagnosis of ingestion of a calciferol-type rodenticide. An attempt to reduce hypercalcaemia by administration of frusemide and glucose/saline infusions was made. One day later calcium had fallen to 3.2 mmol/L (12.9 mg/dl) but urea had elevated, indicating renal damage. The dog was, by this time, very anorexic and was subsequently transferred to the Royal Veterinary College for tests. Renal dysfunction, inappetence and severe weight loss were reported. The animal remained hypercalcaemic, although levels fluctuated.

Aggressive treatment followed, including use of saline infusions, clodronate, frusemide, prednisolone, cimetidine and sucralfate.

The serum calcium levels normalised and stabilised. The intravenous fluids were stopped, but later re-started when the animal became azotaemic and started to vomit and pass diarrhoea. The animal was subsequently discharged with clodronate, cimetidine and sucralfate to be administered over the following week. The animal eventually made a full recovery.

Clinical effects

Signs usually develop within 12–36 hours of ingestion and include depression, lethargy, anorexia, polyuria, polydipsia, profuse vomiting and diarrhoea. Initially, polydipsia may be seen in the absence of any other clinical effects. As the calcium concentrations rise above 12 mg/dl the clinical effects become more severe, this increase usually occurring 24–36 hours post-onset. Effects include severe vomiting, anorexia, constipation, ataxia, arching of the back, muscle spasms, twitching and convulsions. Some animals have pale mucous membranes, dyspnoea and tachypnoea.

Haematemesis and haemorrhagic diarrhoea may occur as a result of calcification in the gastrointestinal tract and pulmonary haemorrhage has also been reported. It is important to recognise that in the absence of positive history such signs could lead to misdiagnosis for anticoagulant rodenticide intoxication.

In severe cases hypercalcaemia, hyperphosphataemia, and deposition of calcium in tissues may cause initial tachycardia, then bradycardia and renal insufficiency characterised by polyuria, azotaemia and hyposthenuria, or renal failure. Leucocytosis is occasionally reported. Cardiac abnormalities may be seen on ECG, commonly shortened QT segment, prolonged PR interval and ventricular arrhythmias. Hypercalcaemic cardiac failure may occur if the serum calcium level exceeds 14 mg/dl. Shock and fulminant pulmonary oedema are common causes of fatality.

Laboratory diagnosis

- A serum calcium concentration higher then 12 mg/dl is characteristic.
- An elevated serum phosphorus level (>5.2 mg/dl) may precede the hypercalcaemia by 12 hours and could serve as an early non-specific indicator.
- Urine specific gravity may range from 1.002–1.006.
- There is elevated BUN (Blood Urea Nitrogen), i.e. >25 mg/dl in severe cases.
- There are elevated creatinine levels in severe cases.
- X-rays (chest/abdominal) may show mineralisation of stomach and upper gastrointestinal tract.
- There are excessive active 1,25-dihydroxycholecalciferol (1,25-dihydroxyvitamin D) metabolites in renal tissue. Analysis is difficult and few laboratories will offer this test routinely.

Unit conversion for calcium – 1 mmol is equivalent to 40.46 mg.

Post-mortem findings

Calcification of soft tissues and blood vessels occurs.

Gross lesions will include petechial haemorrhages, pale streaks in the kidney, pitted mottled kidneys, diffuse haemorrhage of the gastrointestinal tract, roughened raised plaques on the intima of the great vessels and on the surface of the lung and abdominal viscera.

Microscopic lesions include mineralisation of kidney tubules, coronary arteries, gastric mucosa, parietal pleura, pulmonary bronchioles, pancreas and urinary bladder. The renal tubules may be degenerative or necrotic. The liver will show centrilobular congestion. The myocardium may also show evidence of necrosis.

Treatment

Treatment is advised if potentially more than 0.5 mg/kg body weight of calciferol/ cholecalciferol (equivalent to 21 000 IU/kg vitamin D) has been ingested by the dog.

Hence treatment is needed if more than:

- 500 mg/kg body weight of a 0.1% w/w calciferol bait; or
- 25 mg/kg body weight of a 2% w/w calciferol bait; or
- 12.5 mg/kg body weight of a 4% w/w calciferol bait concentrate has been ingested.

Some of the rodenticides that have low concentrations of calciferol or cholecalciferol may contain potentially toxic levels of anticoagulant rodenticides. This should be taken into consideration when deciding whether treatment is necessary following accidental ingestions by dogs (see anticoagulant rodenticide chapter).

Prognosis should be guarded if signs are severe or advanced. Severely poisoned animals usually succumb within 2–5 days of onset of clinical signs

If within 3 hours of ingestion, induce vomiting or perform gastric lavage, and then administer adsorbents.

Emetics:

(a)	Apomorphine	Dose:	0.05 mg/kg body weight i.v. or i.m.; 0.1 mg/kg body weight s.c.
(b)	Xylazine	Dose:	0.2 mg/kg body weight i.v.; 0.5–1 mg/kg body weight i.m. or s.c.
(c)	Ipecacuanha	Dose:	1–2 ml/kg body weight (maximum 20 ml) orally
(d)	Soda crystal.		

Adsorbents:

(a)	Activated charcoal	Dose:	2 g/kg body weight orally
(b)	BCK granules®	Dose:	6–18 g orally 2–3 times daily.

To reduce enterohepatic cycling repeated doses of activated charcoal may be administered. A dose of 2 g/kg body weight can be given every 4 hours until the charcoal appears in the stools.

If there is severe or persistent vomiting then anti-emetics should be administered. If adsorbents have been administered this may reduce efficacy of orally administered anti-emetics. In such cases, parenteral administration is preferable. Either metoclopramide or acepromazine may be used; the latter has a longer duration of action.

(a) Metoclopramide	Dose:	0.5–1 mg/kg body weight orally, s.c. or i.m. every 6–8 hours; 1–2 mg/kg body weight per day by slow i.v. infusion
(b) Acepromazine	Dose:	0.03–0.1 mg/kg body weight i.v., i.m., or s.c. (use lower dose if giving i.v.); 1–3 mg/kg body weight orally.

General care

Ensure adequate hydration and good urine output. In some cases, particularly those where the animal has pre-existing renal insufficiency, dopamine may be necessary to increase renal perfusion (dose: 1–3 µg/kg body weight per minute as constant i.v. infusion).

If possible, the following should be measured/monitored:

- Serum calcium (daily for 3 days, even in asymptomatic cases)
- BUN
- Creatinine
- Urine specific gravity
- ECG.

Diazepam may be given if there is convulsant activity (dose: 0.5 mg/kg body weight i.v., repeated every 10 minutes up to three times if needed).

Administration of cimetidine and/or sucralfate may help prevent damage to the gastric mucosa. Cimetidine reduces gastric acid and pepsin secretions reducing risk of ulcer formation. Sucralfate is an ulcer-coating agent that binds to proteins at ulcer sites, protecting them from further attack by gastric acid and enzymes.

Cimetidine

Dose: 5–10 mg/kg body weight i.v., i.m. or orally every 6–8 hours.

Notes

1. If adsorbents have been administered, then parenteral routes should be employed in the initial stages.
2. If i.v. route is to be used then administer by slow i.v. injection over 30 minutes to reduce risk of hypotension and arrhythmias.
3. If metoclopramide has been used or sucralfate is to be used, then a period of 2 hours should elapse before cimetidine is administered.
4. Adverse effect – cimetidine blocks liver microsomal enzymes and therefore hepatic drug metabolism.

Sucralfate

Dose: in dogs <20 kg body weight 500 mg/dog orally every 6–8 hours; in dogs >20 kg body weight 1 g/dog orally every 6–8 hours.

Notes

1. Where adsorbents have been administered a period of 2 hours should elapse before sucralfate is administered to minimise charcoal binding to drug.
2. If cimetidine is to be used, then sucralfate should be given 2 hours beforehand as it requires an acid environment for maximum efficacy.
3. Ideally sucralfate should be administered on an empty stomach, at least 1 hour prior to food.

Hypercalcaemia

If the animal is hypercalcaemic (level >12 mg/dl), then calciuresis should be attempted using 0.9% saline and administration of frusemide (dose: initial bolus of 5 mg/kg body weight given i.v., followed by a constant rate infusion of 5 mg/kg body weight/hour). The frusemide may also help to prevent onset of pulmonary oedema.

Corticosteroids may be given to limit resorption of calcium from bone, decrease gastrointestinal absorption and to promote renal excretion of calcium (e.g. prednisolone given at a dose of 1–2 mg/kg body weight orally every 12 hours).

Additionally, Salcatonin®, a synthetic salmon calcitonin compound that inhibits bone and intestinal resorption of calcium, may be given. Dose: 4–7 IU/kg body weight s.c., every 6–8 hours. (In the USA this dose would be given every 2–3 hours if needed.) Ideally, administration should be continued until serum calcium stabilises at <12 mg/dl. In some severe cases, this has been required for a period of 3–4 weeks. Unfortunately, anorexia is a common side-effect of this drug, which may prove problematic in dogs that are already anorexic. Dogs tend to regain their appetite some 18 hours after calcitonin administration is ceased.

If available, clodronate, a bisphosphonate that inhibits osteoclast action and suppresses calcium release from bone, may be given. Infusions were used in one past VPIS case. A suggested dose is 400 mg orally every day for 7 days. Clodronate should be given at least 1 hour after food and at least 2 hours either before or after cimetidine administration.

Frusemide and corticosteroids should be continued for 2–4 weeks and, if possible, the serum calcium concentration and BUN should be monitored at 24, 48, 72 hours and 2 weeks *after* cessation of treatment. If the animal is still hypercalcaemic repeated therapy, as above, should be considered.

Notes

1. Frusemide is preferred over thiazide diuretics which can promote hypercalcaemia.
2. Care must be taken to ensure that hypokalaemia does not result from prolonged use of frusemide. This is a potential result of co-administration with corticosteroids. (In some cases, potassium supplementation may be required).
3. The dosage of prednisolone should be tapered off if used for more than 2 weeks, to prevent adrenocortical insufficiency.

Renal insufficiency

If the animal is in renal failure, continuous peritoneal dialysis may be considered.

Long term management

Calcification of soft tissues is irreversible, but its severity may be limited by preventing access to sunlight and restricting calcium intake. Diets high in fluid and salt and low in calcium and devoid of milk and dairy products are strongly advocated.

References and further reading

VPIS (London) past cases up to 97/37546.

Buronfosse F, Buronfosse T and Berny P (1998). Cholecalciferol poisoning in dogs. *Veterinary and Human Toxicology* **40(3)**, 173.

Cumming C (1991). Suspected vitamin D rodenticide poisoning in a dog. *Veterinary Record* **128(5)**, 600.

Dorman DC (1990). Anticoagulant, cholecalciferol, and bromethalin-based rodenticides. *Veterinary Clinics of North America: Small Animal Practice* **20(2)**, 339–352.

El Bahri L *et al.* (1990). Poisoning in dogs by vitamin D₃ containing rodenticides. *Compendium on Continuing Education* **12**, 1414–1417.

Fooshee SK and Forrester SD (1990). Hypercalcaemia secondary to cholecalciferol rodenticide toxicosis in two dogs. *Journal of the American Veterinary Medical Association* **196(8)**, 1265–1268.

Gunther R *et al.* (1988). Toxicity of a vitamin D₃ rodenticide to dogs. *Journal of the American Veterinary Medical Association* **193(2)**, 211–214.

Nesbitt T (1988). Comments on toxicity of a vitamin D₃ rodenticide. *Journal of the American Veterinary Medical Association* **193(7)**, 757.

Ross LA (1988). Comments on toxicity of a vitamin D₃ rodenticide. *Journal of the American Veterinary Medical Association* **193(7)**, 757.

Studdert VP *et al.* (1990). Toxicity of cholecalciferol-containing rodenticides for dogs and cats. *Australian Veterinary Journal* **67(6)**, 218.

Talcott PA *et al.* (1991). Accidental ingestion of a cholecalciferol containing rodent bait in a dog. *Veterinary and Human Toxicology* **33(3)**, 252–256.

Cannabis / Marihuana / Hashish

The agent

Cannabis is the collective term for all psychoactive substances derived from the dried leaves and flowers of the plant *Cannabis sativa* or hemp. Marihuana refers to any part of the plant used to induce effects and hashish is the dried resin from the flower tops.

Occurrence of poisoning incidences

Since 1992 the VPIS centre in London has received approximately 10 enquiries per year regarding ingestion of cannabis, marihuana or hashish. All of these cases have involved dogs. Some involved sniffer dogs owned by the police or Customs who had inadvertently ingested the drugs during training or normal work. In all cases, the animals have shown effects as a result of exposure but all made a complete recovery.

Toxicity

In animals, ingestion is the common route of exposure, although apocryphal cases of inhalational poisoning occurring in dogs due to their owners smoking cannabis have been reported to the VPIS London centre.

Often the preparations that are obtained 'off the street' are impure and other effects may be seen due to other constituents.

According to the literature:

- A minimum lethal dose of more than 3 mg/kg body weight for dogs is quoted.
- Toxic doses are quoted in the range 50–100 mg/kg body weight for the plant.
- Fatal cases would generally be unlikely to occur.

In the experience of the VPISLn:

- No fatal cases reported.
- However, all cases referred have exhibited clinical effects.
- Recovery can take up to 4 days.

Mechanism of toxicity

The plant may contain between 1 and 6% by weight delta-9-tetrahydro-cannabinol (THC), which is the principal toxic constituent. THC is most concentrated in the leaves and flower tops of the plant. In 'recreational' use in man, marihuana is smoked or ingested in doses of 5–10 mg of THC. In man, about 10–50% of an inhaled dose is absorbed and about 6% of an ingested dose. Cannabis appears to have similar effects in dogs as in man.

The exact mechanism of action of the THC and other metabolites is not clear. The actions may be linked to changing levels of biogenic amines in the CNS.

Kinetics and metabolism

Absorption and onset of effects is usually rapid following both ingestion or inhalation. The THC undergoes enterohepatic recirculation, resulting in sustained levels and production of a variety of active metabolites. 6 to 20% of an ingested dose may reach the systemic circulation. THC is highly lipophilic.

Clinical effects

Onset of effects is usually within 1–3 hours, and total recovery usually within 24–72 hours. In some VPIS cases, complete recovery has taken 4 days.

Effects usually include weakness, ataxia (often pronounced in the hind limbs), drowsiness, dilated pupils, nystagmus, photophobia, tachycardia, urinary and faecal incontinence, and hyperaesthesia. Behavioural changes occur including aggression, agitation and barking. It is possible that the animals hallucinate. Dogs appear to develop a heightened sense of smell and hearing and may obsessively investigate sights, sounds and odours. The animals may later develop deep depression, stupor, bradycardia, and analgesia.

There may also be conjunctival injection, vomiting, excessive salivation, muscle weakness, hypotension, increased appetite, hyperthermia, hyperventilation, shaking, twitching and, rarely, convulsions.

Post-mortem findings

No findings definitively attributed to cannabis or marihuana have been determined.

Treatment

Treatment is recommended for any amount. Emesis may be induced within 1 hour of the ingestion, provided the animal is asymptomatic. Emetics may not always be effective, as THC can have an anti-emetic action.

Use of absorbents is also recommended. Repeated doses (every 4 hours) may be effective in reducing levels as the THC undergoes enterohepatic recirculation.

Emetics:

(a) Apomorphine	Dose:	0.05 mg/kg body weight i.v. or i.m.; 0.1 mg/kg body weight s.c.
(b) Xylazine	Dose:	0.2 mg/kg body weight i.v.; 0.5–1 mg/kg body weight i.m. or s.c.
(c) Ipecacuanha	Dose:	1–2 ml/kg body weight (maximum 20 ml) orally
(d) Soda crystal.		

Adsorbents:

(a) Activated charcoal	Dose:	2 g/kg body weight orally.

Repeat 4-hourly, if required, until charcoal appears in the stools.

(b) BCK granules®	Dose:	6–18 g orally 2–3 times daily.

Treatment thereafter is largely supportive. A minimum observation period of 2 hours post-exposure is recommended.

Sedation using diazepam may be given where necessary. Diazepam dose: 0.5 mg/kg body weight i.v. repeated every 10 minutes up to three times if needed.

Where possible, the animal should be kept in a relatively quiet dark environment. Body temperature should be monitored, as provision of artificial/supplemental heat may be necessary. Intravenous fluid may be required in animals that become hypotensive.

Investigative

THC can be detected in both blood and urine and such tests can be used to confirm exposure.

References and further reading

VPIS (London) past cases up to 97/114004.

Dumonceaux GA and Beasley VR (1990). Emergency treatments for police dogs used for illicit drug detection. *Journal of the American Veterinary Medical Association* **197(2)**, 185–187.

Frost RC (1983). Marijuana toxaemia. *Veterinary Record* **112**, 441.

Frye FL (1968). Acute cannabis intoxication in a pup. *Journal of the American Veterinary Medical Association* **152(5)**, 472.

Godbold JC et al. (1979). Acute oral marijuana poisoning in a dog. *Journal of the American Veterinary Medical Association* **175(10)**, 1101–1102.

Godwin RLG (1992). Unusual poisoning in a dog. *Veterinary Record* **130**, 335–336.

Henney SN and Coleman MJ (1984). Canine cannabis intoxication. *Veterinary Record* **114**, 436.

Jones DL (1978). A case of canine cannabis ingestion. *New Zealand Veterinary Journal* **26**, 135–136.

Kisseberth WC and Trammel HL (1990). Illicit and abused drugs. *Veterinary Clinics of North America: Small Animal Practice* **20(2)**, 405–418.

Schwartz RH (1989). Comments on cannabis intoxication in pets. *Veterinary and Human Toxicology* **31(3)**, 262.

Schwartz RH and Riddile M (1985). Marijuana intoxication in pets. *Journal of the American Veterinary Medical Association* **187(3)**, 206.

Silverman J (1974). Possible hashish intoxication in a dog. *Journal of the American Animal Hospital Association* **10(5)**, 517–519.

Thursby-Pelham C (1996). Peculiar drug poisonings in pets. *In Practice* **18(10)**, 478–487.

Valentine J (1992). Unusual poisoning in a dog. *Veterinary Record* **130**, 307.

Carbamate insecticides

Type of product

Carbamate insecticides are widely used as garden and household pesticides, and in agriculture.

Presentation

Formulations include liquids, sprays and powders, which may be used as supplied or diluted; liquid preparations often contain organic solvents. Shampoos, aqueous and alcoholic lotions are also used as human pedicullicides and scabicides.

Carbaryl and propoxur are used in veterinary medicine for the control of fleas.

Many agricultural preparations contain carbamates in combination with organophosphates.

Substances covered include *aldicarb, bendiocarb, carbaryl, carbofuran, propoxur*.

See separate entry for methiocarb.

Occurrence of poisoning incidences

Since 1992 the VPIS London centre has received between 20 and 60 enquiries per year about the various carbamates. The majority of cases reported involve bendiocarb-containing ant killers and methiocarb slug baits. No fatal cases involving bendiocarb, carbaryl, carbofuran or propoxur have been reported to the VPISLn, although some animals have exhibited severe clinical effects.

Toxicity

Toxic doses for many of the carbamates in dogs have not been established.

According to the literature:

Aldicarb

- The LD_{50} for aldicarb in dogs is 5–10 mg/kg body weight.

Carbaryl

- The LD_{50} for carbaryl in dogs is 250–795 mg/kg body weight.

Carbofuran

* The LD$_{50}$ of carbofuran in dogs is 15–19 mg/kg body weight.

In the experience of VPISLn:

Aldicarb

* One fatal canine case has been reported. A Border Collie ingested an unknown quantity of an agricultural insecticide containing aldicarb. Within 2 hours the animal had collapsed, and displayed excessive salivation, pin-point pupils, tremors and fitting. Emesis was induced, and the animal given atropine, diazepam and diuretics, but died shortly afterwards (VPISLn case 92/9957).

Bendiocarb

* Many cases of ingestion of bendiocarb-containing products have been reported. However, none have had a fatal outcome. Those involving ingestion of ant or woodlice killers, where bendiocarb is usually present in concentrations of about 0.5%, rarely exhibit more than gastrointestinal discomfort. Ingestion of products intended for agricultural use has resulted in ataxia, tremors, fitting, salivation and constricted pupils, with skin irritation evident after dermal exposures. With symptomatic and supportive care all made a rapid recovery.

Carbofuran

* Two canine cases with significant clinical effects have been reported. Both had salivation, vomiting, tremors, incoordination and pyrexia. With symptomatic care both animals made a good, if slow, recovery (VPISLn cases 87/22286 and 94/8893).

Mechanism of toxicity

Like organophosphates, carbamates bind to and inhibit acetylcholinesterase. This results in accumulation of the neurotransmitter acetylcholine and activation of nicotinic receptors at skeletal muscle end plates, autonomic ganglia and within the CNS, and of muscarinic receptors at smooth muscle myoneural junctions and exocrine and endocrine secretory systems. Therefore, both nicotinic and muscarinic effects occur, although nicotinic receptors rapidly become desensitised. Myopathy is thought to be secondary to excessive acetylcholine stimulation of muscle.

Compared with the phosphorylated enzyme that results from organophosphate poisoning, the carbamylated acetylcholinesterase is less stable, and spontaneous reversal to the carbamate and acetylcholinesterase occurs. As a result, the effects resulting from carbamate poisoning tend to be of much shorter duration compared with those of organophosphate poisoning and use of cholinesterase reactivators (such as pralidoxime) is unnecessary.

Atropine acts as a non-competitive antagonist by blocking the effect of the muscarinic receptors on target organs.

Kinetics and metabolism

Carbamates are generally highly lipophilic and may be absorbed from the gastrointestinal tract, through the skin and following exposure to high concentrations via the lungs. They are rapidly excreted.

Clinical effects

Onset of effects is usually from within 30 minutes to 3 hours.

Mild to moderate effects normally include salivation, bronchial hypersecretion, ataxia, diarrhoea, constricted pupils, muscle fasciculation, tremors and twitching, weakness, shaking, hyperaesthesia, pyrexia, restlessness and urinary incontinence.

In severe cases collapse, bradycardia, respiratory depression, convulsions, cyanosis and coma may occur.

Myopathy occurs rarely following recovery.

Carbamates do not cause the delayed neurotoxicity observed after some organophosphate poisonings. This is due to the lack of ageing with carbamates.

Laboratory findings

These are generally non-specific and include increased packed cell volume (PCV), raised serum aspartate transaminase (AST) and creatinine phosphokinase (CPK). Elevated serum amylase may be noted.

Post-mortem findings

There are no characteristic lesions observed in carbamate insecticide poisoned animals. Pulmonary changes may be observed, including bronchoconstriction, increased bronchial secretions and pulmonary oedema. Pancreatitis may be present.

Treatment

If the ingestion has occurred within 2 hours, vomiting may be induced, or perform gastric lavage and then administer adsorbents.

Emetics:

(a) Apomorphine	Dose:	0.05 mg/kg body weight i.v. or i.m.; 0.1 mg/kg body weight s.c.
(b) Xylazine	Dose:	0.2 mg/kg body weight i.v.; 0.5–1 mg/kg body weight i.m. or s.c.

(c)	Ipecacuanha	Dose:	1–2 ml/kg body weight (maximum 20 ml) orally
(d)	Soda crystal.		

Adsorbents:

(a)	Activated charcoal	Dose:	2 g/kg body weight orally
(b)	BCK granules®	Dose:	6–18 g orally 2–3 times daily.

If there is a risk of dermal exposure the animal should be thoroughly washed with a mild detergent.

Further management is largely symptomatic; in particular, body temperature should be maintained, and blood gases and electrolytes monitored and corrected. Rehydration may be required.

If sedation is required then diazepam may be given. Dose: 0.5 mg/kg body weight i.v. repeated every 10 minutes up to three times if needed.

Atropine should be given to reverse cholinergic effects. Dose: 0.2–2 mg/kg body weight (one-quarter of the dose given i.v. and the remainder s.c. or i.m.), repeated as required (usually every 45–90 minutes initially). Large doses may be required for effect.

Atropine has no effect on nicotinic receptors and will not counteract skeletal muscle tremors, weakness or neuromuscular paralysis. However, effects from carbamates such as methiocarb are generally short-lived and cholinesterase reactivators such as pralidoxime are not required. In cases of poisoning with an organophosphate-carbamate mixture, pralidoxime should be given if required (see Organophosphate chapter).

Contra-indicated drugs

Phenothiazine sedatives and succinylcholine should be avoided because of the neuromuscular blocking activity, since they will exacerbate the toxicity of carbamates. Antibiotics such as aminoglycosides (e.g. streptomycin, gentamicin, neomycin, kanamycin), polypeptides (e.g. polymixin A and B) and clindamycin should also be avoided, since they may have neuromuscular blocking effects. Benzodiazepines, opioids and barbiturates should be used cautiously because of their CNS depressant effects.

Laboratory investigations

Cholinesterase activity determination may be considered. It is advised that whole blood from unaffected animals should also be submitted as a control. Although not a uniformly reliable indicator, a decrease of 50% or more of normal activity generally indicates significant inhibition and in many cases the cholinesterase activity is less than 25% of normal. In cases of carbamate poisoning, whole blood samples must be rapidly collected, frozen and transported to the laboratory because of spontaneous reactivation of cholinesterase.

References and further reading

VPIS (London) past cases up to 98/12409.

Fikes JD (1990). Organophosphate and carbamate insecticides. *Veterinary Clinics of North America: Small Animal Practice* **20(2)**, 353–367.

McEntree K *et al.* (1994). Acute polymyopathy after carbamate poisoning in a dog. *Veterinary Record* **134**, 88–89.

Talcott PA and Dorman DC (1997). Pesticide exposures in companion animals. *Veterinary Medicine* **92(2)**, 167–181.

Chocolate / Theobromine

The agent

Theobromine is a methylxanthine occurring as the major alkaloid in chocolate and cocoa powder. Chocolate is derived from the roasted seeds of the plant *Theobroma cacao*. Cocoa solids account for some 30–70% of chocolate.

Presentation

The concentration of theobromine from various sources commonly implicated in poisoning incidents is shown below. Chocolate also contains a small amount of caffeine (also a methylxanthine).

Source	Theobromine content per g of product
White chocolate	0.009 mg (9 ppm)
Drinking chocolate (dry)	0.5 mg
Milk chocolate	1.5–2.2 mg
Plain chocolate	4.5–16 mg
Cocoa powder	5.3–26 mg
Cocoa beans	11–43 mg
Cocoa shell mulches	14–30 mg

Occurrence of poisoning incidences

Since 1992 the VPIS has received a significant number of enquiries concerning theobromine intoxication in dogs, resulting from a variety of sources. In 1997, 53 enquiries were received, representing some 1.6% of the total enquiry number. Several deaths have been reported.

Toxicity

According to the literature:

- Fatal doses of theobromine for dogs are quoted in the range 90–250 mg/kg body weight.
- A dose of 130 mg/kg was lethal in a dog.
- The LD_{50} is quoted as 300 mg/kg body weight.
- 12 mg/kg caused no visible ill effects.

In the experience of the VPISLn:

- Several fatal cases reported.
- These usually result from ingestion of cocoa powder or cocoa shell mulches.

Mechanism of toxicity

Methylxanthine intoxication in dogs produces a characteristic picture of CNS stimulation with cardiac and respiratory hyperactivity. Theobromine directly stimulates both the myocardium and the CNS.

Methylxanthines exert their effect by a variety of mechanisms. They competitively antagonise cellular adenosine receptors, resulting in CNS stimulation, vasoconstriction and tachycardia. They also inhibit cellular phosphodiesterase, causing an increase in cyclic AMP, increased release of catecholamines, increased entry of calcium and inhibition of calcium sequestration by the sarcoplasmic reticulum, causing increased muscular contractility in both skeletal and cardiac muscle. Theobromine also competitively inhibits benzodiazepine receptors in the brain.

Kinetics and metabolism

In dogs, absorption is slow compared with that in man. It is reported to take some 10 hours to be fully absorbed. Theobromine is metabolised in the liver by microsomal mixed-function oxidases, N-demethylation and conjugation, with the products being excreted in urine. As the metabolic products are alkaline they are more rapidly excreted if the urine is acidified. Theobromine also undergoes enterohepatic recirculation.

Clinical effects

Onset of clinical effects is generally within 24 hours, usually within 4 hours. Duration of effects may be as long as 72 hours.

Vomiting, abdominal tenderness, polydipsia, haematemesis, restlessness, excitability, hyperactivity, mild hypertension, salivation, diuresis, ataxia and tachycardia (sometimes bradycardia) are commonly encountered clinical effects.

In severe cases, there may be muscle rigidity, tachypnoea, diarrhoea, urinary incontinence, haematuria, cyanosis, hyperthermia, tremors, convulsions and arrhythmias (classically ventricular premature beats). Occasionally, renal dysfunction has been reported.

Fatal outcomes are usually associated with severe convulsions and acute circulatory failure.

Post-mortem findings

Often gross evidence of chocolate or cocoa in the gastrointestinal tract is a finding.

Hyperaemia of the gastric and proximal duodenal mucosa, diffuse congestion and hyperaemia of the kidneys, liver, spleen and pancreas, and petechial and ecchymotic haemorrhaging in thymus have all been commonly reported. Microscopic changes reported include presence of pyknotic nuclei in distal renal tubular epithelium, and cytoplasmic hyaline droplets, with pyknosis and karyorrhexis in epithelium of renal convoluted tubules.

In one fatal case involving ingestion of cocoa post-mortem revealed diffuse pulmonary congestion.

Treatment

Treatment is recommended for ingestions of more than 20 mg/kg body weight of theobromine or equivalent.

In asymptomatic animals, both an emetic and adsorbents should be given if the ingestion occurred within the previous 3 hours. Where the animals are hyperactive or excitable, emesis is best avoided and adsorbents alone given.

Repeated doses of adsorbents may be useful in enhancing elimination, as theobromine undergoes enterohepatic recirculation

Emetics:

(a) Apomorphine	Dose:	0.05 mg/kg body weight i.v. or i.m.; 0.1 mg/kg body weight s.c.	
(b) Xylazine	Dose:	0.2 mg/kg body weight i.v.; 0.5–1 mg/kg body weight i.m. or s.c.	
(c) Ipecacuanha	Dose:	1–2 ml/kg body weight (maximum 20 ml) orally	
(d) Soda crystal.			

Adsorbents:

(a) Activated charcoal	Dose:	2 g/kg body weight orally. Repeat 4 hourly, if required, until charcoal appears in the stools.	
(b) BCK granules	Dose:	6–18 g orally two or three times daily.	

If there is severe or persistent vomiting then anti-emetics should be administered. If adsorbents have been administered, this may reduce efficacy of orally administered anti-emetics. In such cases, parenteral administration is preferable. Either metoclopramide or acepromazine may be used; the latter has a longer duration of action.

(a) Metoclopramide	Dose:	0.5–1 mg/kg body weight orally, s.c. or i.m. every 6–8 hours; 1–2 mg/kg body weight per day by slow i.v. infusion	
(b) Acepromazine	Dose:	0.03–0.1 mg/kg body weight i.v., i.m., or s.c. (use lower dose if giving i.v.); 1–3 mg/kg body weight orally.	

Diazepam may be administered if the animal is hyperactive or has convulsions. Where this proves ineffective, owing to the blocking of benzodiazepine receptors, then use of barbiturates such as pentobarbitone may be considered.

Doses recommended:

(a) Diazepam   0.5 mg/kg body weight i.v. repeated every 10 minutes
                       up to three times if needed.

(b) Pentobarbitone   3–15 mg/kg body weight i.v. slowly until effect.

Monitor temperature and ensure adequate hydration. If possible, monitor ECG
and renal function.

Some authors have suggested catheterisation of the animal to prevent re-
absorption of theobromine across the bladder mucosa.

Where tachycardia is severe or other arrhythmias are present some authors
suggest use of propranolol, metoprolol or lidocaine.

Doses recommended:

(a) Lidocaine   1–4 mg i.v. over 2–3 minutes as a loading dose,
                       followed by infusion of 0.1% solution at a rate of
                       25–75 μg/kg body weight per minute.

(b) Propranolol   0.02–0.15 mg/kg body weight i.v. over 2–3 minutes or
                       0.1 mg/kg body weight orally every 8 hours

(c) Metoprolol   0.04–0.06 mg/kg body weight by slow i.v. injection
                       every 8 hours.

Notes

1. Use of propranolol may slow renal excretion of theobromine.
2. Care should be taken when using all of the above three drugs as severe
   hypotension may result owing to unopposed alpha-adrenergic effects.

Where the animal is bradycardic, atropine may be given. Dose: 0.02–0.04 mg/kg
body weight i.v.

Investigative

Theobromine may be measured in blood samples.

References and further reading

VPIS (London) past cases up to 98/36540.

Drolet R, Arendt TD and Stowe CM (1984). Cocoa bean shell poisoning in a dog. *Journal of the American Veterinary Medical Association* **185(8)**, 902.

Decker RA and Myers GH (1972). Theobromine poisoning. *Journal of the American Veterinary Medical Association* **161(2)**, 198–199.

Glauberg A and Blumenthal HP (1983). Chocolate poisoning in the dog. *Journal of the American Animal Hospital Association* **19(2)**, 246–248.

Hovda LR and Kingston RL (1994). Cocoa bean mulch poisoning in dogs (abstract 76). *Veterinary and Human Toxicology* **36(4)**, 357.

Kisseberth WC and Trammel HL (1990). Illicit and abused drugs. *Veterinary Clinics of North America: Small Animal Practice* **20(2)**, 405–418.

Owens JG and Dorman DC (1997). Drug poisoning in small animals. *Veterinary Medicine* **92(2)**, 149–156.

Sutton RH (1981). Cocoa poisoning in a dog. *Veterinary Record* **109(25–26)**, 563–564.

Strachan ER and Bennett A (1994). Theobromine poisoning in dogs. *Veterinary Record* **134(11)**, 284.

Corticosteroids

Type of product

This is a large group of drugs used for a variety of disorders including allergic and immune-mediated diseases, cardiogenic and septic shock, trauma and oedema.

Presentation

Corticosteroids are available as tablets, syrups, parenteral preparations, and creams or ointments for dermal application.

Occurrence of poisoning incidences

Every year the VPIS receives a number of enquires regarding the potential toxicity of corticosteroid preparations in domestic pets. Most of these enquiries concern dogs and usually involve accidental ingestion of preparations intended for human use. No serious cases have been reported.

Recommended dosage

This varies, depending on the specific drug and the indication.

Toxicity

These drugs are considered of low toxicity in acute overdose.

Clinical effects

There are usually none, but vomiting and diarrhoea may occur, particularly following ingestion of a cream or ointment.

Treatment

No treatment is necessary, even for very substantial ingestions.

Reference

VPIS (London) past cases up to 98/134769.

Cotoneaster species

The plant

Common species are *Cotoneaster horizontalis*, *Cotoneaster pyracantha* and *Cotoneaster simonsii*. The plants belong to the Rosaceae family.

Cotoneaster is an evergreen or deciduous low-growing shrub or tree with horizontally growing stems and branches that may grow to heights of about 5 m. It is commonly encountered in public parks and private gardens.

The plant has small, oval, green leaves, which are dark and shiny on the upper side and pale on the underside. The plant bears small white or pale pink flowers from May to August and an abundance of round, bright red berries from June or July onwards. There are species where the berries are a white or yellow colour. The berries are usually about 5–8 mm in diameter, have a mealy pulp and contain up to three seeds. Berries may remain on the plant until winter.

Occurrence of poisoning incidences

Since the launch of the VPIS, the centre in London has received a small number of enquiries each year regarding ingestion of cotoneaster berries by dogs. No fatal cases in dogs have been reported, and many of the cases reported to the VPIS have been asymptomatic.

Toxicity

Exposures usually occur in gardens or in woodland areas, often when the animals are exercising. In general, the plant is considered to be of low toxicity, although if huge quantities were ingested then clinical effects might occur. One paper in the literature describes how an 18 kg dog was starved for 24 hours and then fed blended cotoneaster fruit at a dosing of 10 g/kg body weight mixed with its normal feed. No clinical effects were observed in the following 24-hour period (Tidwell *et al.*, 1970).

Mechanism of toxicity

Cotoneaster species contain cyanogenic glycosides. Prunasin is found in the bark, leaves and flowers, and both prunasin and amygdalin are found in the fruit. The glycosides in the fruit appear to be concentrated in the fleshy part rather than in the stone. The concentration of both prunasin and amygdalin varies greatly from species to species, and varies according to the ripeness of the fruit.

Clinical effects

The principal effects are those of gastrointestinal upset. In the cases reported to the VPISLn the clinical effects commonly observed are salivation, vomiting and diarrhoea, which may be bloody. Excessive fluid loss may lead to dehydration. Hypothermia has been reported in one VPISLn case (93/111269).

Treatment

Gastric decontamination using gastric lavage or emesis is not necessary as the berries are of low toxicity and vomiting usually occurs spontaneously. Use of metoclopramide may be considered if vomiting is severe.

Metoclopramide dose: 0.5–1 mg/kg body weight orally, s.c. or i.m. every 6–8 hours; 1–2 mg/kg body weight per day by slow i.v. infusion.

Ensure that the animal is well hydrated. Warming methods (e.g. a heat pad) may be necessary for hypothermia.

References

VPIS (London) past cases up to 97/139666.

Tidwell RH *et al.* (1970). A study of the cyanogenetic content and toxicity of the fruit of selected species of *Cotoneaster*. *Economic Botany* **24**, 47–50.

Cyanoacrylate adhesives

Type of product

Rapid setting adhesives for household use. So-called 'superglues' are usually cyanoacrylate adhesives.

Occurrence of poisoning incidences

Since the launch of the VPIS in 1992, up to 15 enquiries per year have been received about canine exposures to cyanoacrylate glues. In about one-third of these, the exposures were either to the eye or to the ear, as a result of mistaken administration by the owners.

Toxicity

Cyanoacrylate glues are non-toxic by ingestion.

On setting heat may be produced, which can cause local irritation. There is also the risk of obstruction if large, solid lumps are swallowed. Cyanoacrylate glues in the ear can cause occlusion of the ear canal and may be difficult to remove. These glues are often applied to the ear or eye, being mistaken for ear or eye drops.

Clinical effects

Ingestion

Ingestion may result in localised irritation, vomiting, 'coughing' and salivation. It is very difficult to swallow cyanoacrylate glues as they set very quickly. Occasionally the glue may adhere strongly to the gums, teeth and tongue. Theoretically, obstruction could occur if large lumps of solidified glue are swallowed.

Eye

Applications to the eyes of dogs has resulted in apparent pain and irritation. Any lumps of glue stuck under the eyelid may abrade the cornea. Occasionally the eyelids of dogs have been glued together.

Ear

Applications into the ear canal cause apparent pain, burning and ulceration of the ear canal. Occlusion of the ear canal may result.

Skin

Dermal exposures usually result in mild irritation only, although animals may damage skin further in their attempts to remove glue that has adhered to the skin.

Treatment

Ingestion

Oral fluids may be given. Lumps of glue that are firmly stuck to the teeth or lining of the mouth should not be removed. Saliva lifts and removes the glue within 12–48 hours. However, there is the risk of choking if large lumps detach. Any loosened lumps of glue should be gently removed.

Eye

The affected eye should be irrigated with saline or water and the eyelids separated surgically if necessary. Management is otherwise supportive. Use of commercially available 'superglue' removers is not recommended as these contain solvents, which may further irritate the cornea.

Ear

The ear should be irrigated with warm water or saline. Manual removal of the glue should be attempted where possible, although complete removal of all the glue may not be possible at once and may have to be achieved over several days. Use of commercially available 'superglue' removers is not recommended. Topical antibiotics may be needed to minimise the risk of infection.

Skin

Where possible, the affected areas should be washed and loose glue particles should be detached. If necessary, areas that remain glued should be bandaged or the animal collared to prevent damage through self-grooming.

Reference

VPIS (London) past cases up to 97/167648.

Daffodil

The plant

Common species are: *Narcissus pseudonarcissus* (Wild daffodil, Lent lily) and *Narcissus poeticus* (Poet's daffodil, Pheasant's eye daffodil).

These plants belong to the Amaryllidaceae family and *Narcissus* genus.

They are perennial plants, which grow from a fleshy white bulb that is surrounded by a dark flaky skin. They have long, erect, green leaves and a pale green hollow stem, which when broken exudes a clear sticky sap. The fruit is a small, green capsule filled with minute black seeds. The plant flowers from March to April with characteristic white or yellow trumpet-shaped flowers. They grow both wild and cultivated.

Occurrence of poisoning incidences

Since the launch of the VPIS, the centre in London has received a small number of enquiries each year regarding ingestion of daffodils. Most of these enquiries involve dogs. All but three have developed clinical effects. Four cases with severe poisoning have been reported, of which one died and one was euthanased. Effects have ranged from mild gastritis to severe dehydration.

Toxicity

In most cases, it is the bulbs that have been ingested by dogs but poisoning has been reported following ingestion of daffodil flowers. Mild poisoning is possible if water in which cut specimens have been standing is drunk.

According to the literature:

- A portion of one bulb may be toxic or lethal to small animals.
- Lethal dose is 15 g of bulbs.

In the experience of the VPISLn:

- A 4-month-old Cocker Spaniel ate 12 flower heads. It developed profuse vomiting and drowsiness 1 hour post-ingestion. The animal made a spontaneous recovery (VPISLn case 86/9476).
- An 8-month-old Golden Retriever ate an unknown quantity of bulbs. Within 3 hours the animal had weakness, pale mucous membranes, bradycardia, hypothermia, hyperglycaemia and vomiting. The animal was treated with i.v. fluids, dexamethasone, insulin, adrenaline and diazepam and recovered (VPISLn case 92/22188).

- A 6-year-old cross-bred dog ingested an unknown number of bulbs. It presented with severe abdominal pain, hypersalivation, pale mucous membranes, and watery diarrhoea. Investigations revealed elevated urea and creatinine. The animal deteriorated rapidly and was euthanased at the owner's request (VPISLn case 93/105033).

Mechanism of toxicity

Daffodils contain alkaloids and glycosides, which are responsible for the clinical effects observed. These agents are present in all parts of the plant but are most concentrated in the bulbs. The alkaloids are all phenanthridine derivatives and include narcissine, narciclasine, galanthamine and lycorine of which lycorine, occurs at the highest concentration. The glycosides include scillitoxin. Calcium oxalate crystals are also present. Lycorine and the alkaloids have irritant, emetic and purgative actions and calcium oxalate acts as a mechanical irritant.

Clinical effects

Onset from 15 minutes to 24 hours has been reported to VPISLn.

Common clinical effects include vomiting, diarrhoea, abdominal tenderness, anorexia, salivation, pyrexia, lethargy and pale mucous membranes. In severe cases following ingestion of large amounts, ataxia, collapse, hypothermia, hypotension, bradycardia, severe abdominal pain, hyperglycaemia and dehydration would be anticipated. Tremors or convulsions are theoretically possible. Deaths are rare.

Pruritis and erythema may occur following contact with the sap.

Post-mortem findings

Findings are non-specific. There may be evidence of severe gastroenteritis and plant material present in the gastrointestinal lumen.

Treatment

Vomiting may be induced in the unlikely event that it has not already occurred and if the animal is presented within 2 hours of ingestion. Alternatively, gastric lavage may be considered.

Emetics:

(a)	Apomorphine	Dose:	0.05 mg/kg body weight i.v. or i.m.; 0.1 mg/kg body weight s.c.
(b)	Xylazine	Dose:	0.2 mg/kg body weight i.v.; 0.5–1 mg/kg body weight i.m. or s.c.
(c)	Ipecacuanha	Dose:	1–2 ml/kg body weight (maximum 20 ml) orally
(d)	Soda crystal.		

If there is severe or persistent vomiting, metoclopramide may be given. Dose: 0.5–1 mg/kg body weight orally, s.c. or i.m. every 6–8 hours; 1–2 mg/kg body weight per day by slow i.v. infusion.

Intravenous fluid support should be given to maintain hydration.

Reference

VPIS (London) past cases up to 97/47994.

Diclofenac sodium

Type of product

Diclofenac sodium is a non-steroidal anti-inflammatory drug (NSAID) with antipyretic and analgesic activity.

Presentation

Diclofenac is available in the UK as a 'prescription only' medicine for humans, with indications for use in the management of pain and inflammation in rheumatic diseases, gout, musculoskeletal disorders, and for management of postoperative pain and dental pain. It is sold under various brand names in tablet, capsule, gel and suppository preparations. A liquid preparation for injection is also available.

Some tablet preparations contain diclofenac in combination with misoprostol. The rationale for the formulation of this compound preparation is given below.

The dose of diclofenac sodium in tablet and capsule preparations varies but is commonly 25 mg, 50 mg, 75 mg and 100 mg. Some of these are modified release preparations. Those in combination usually contain 200 μg of misoprostol.

Suppository preparations contain 12.5 mg, 25 mg, 50 mg. or 100 mg of diclofenac sodium. Gel preparations contain the diethylammonium salt of diclofenac in strengths equivalent to 1 g diclofenac sodium per 100 g of product.

The preparation for injection contains 25 mg/ml of diclofenac sodium. It is available in 3 ml ampoules.

Occurrence of poisoning incidences

Ingestions of diclofenac by dogs feature regularly in the enquiries made to the VPIS London centre. Since 1993, between 10 and 32 enquiries per year have been received, with almost all of these cases occurring in dogs. These enquiries represent approximately 0.8% of the total enquiries made. Only one fatal case has been reported to the VPIS London centre. However, many dogs are presented to veterinary practices with moderate clinical effects.

Recommended dosage

Diclofenac is not licensed for veterinary use in the UK.

Toxicity

It is well known that dogs are particularly sensitive to the propionic acid group of NSAIDs, but there is less documentation about phenylacetic acid-derived NSAIDs such as diclofenac sodium. It would appear that this group of NSAIDs is likely to cause dogs to develop severe gastric ulceration and intestinal irritation, as does the propionic acid-derived variety. It would also appear that there is a risk of renal impairment or failure in dogs who receive high doses.

According to the literature:

- LD_{50} in dogs is quoted as 59 mg/kg body weight.

In the experience of the VPISLn:

- Doses as high as 90 mg/kg body weight have not resulted in any clinical effects. However, single doses of 30 mg/kg body weight or more frequently result in mild gastrointestinal effects, such as vomiting and diarrhoea.
- One dog received a dose of 2.5 mg/kg body weight and developed vomiting and abdominal tenderness over 24 hours. The animal was treated with ranitidine and metoclopramide and recovered (VPISLn case 97/9205).
- A 6-month-old Whippet ate 50 mg/kg body weight. Within 8 hours the dog was depressed and had severe gastritis and diarrhoea. With i.v. fluid support and cimetidine, metoclopramide, sucralfate and ampicillin the animal made a slow recovery (VPISLn case 95/61427).
- A 9-year-old Cocker Spaniel received a total dose of 38.5 mg/kg body weight in divided doses over a period of 4 days. The animal was presented with melena, vomiting, pale mucous membranes and dehydration. The animal was treated with i.v. fluids, cimetidine, sucralfate and antibiotics and made a slow recovery (VPISLn case 95/96911).
- A Doberman puppy accidentally ate a dose equivalent to 800 mg/kg body weight. The animal was presented with haematuria, bloody diarrhoea, anaemia and polydipsia. Laboratory investigation indicated renal impairment. The animal received i.v. fluids, steroids, cimetidine and antibiotics but died (VPISLn case 96/68838).

Mechanism of toxicity

Like other NSAIDs, diclofenac sodium competitively inhibits the cyclo-oxygenase step of prostaglandin synthesis. Such inhibition and subsequent reduction in levels of PGI_2 and PGE_2 can account for the major effects seen in poisoning cases.

In the gastrointestinal tract, prostaglandins have a cytoprotective function as they control production of gastric acid, stimulate secretion of mucous and bicarbonate by the gastric epithelium and maintain mucosal blood flow by causing vasodilatation. Deficiency will result in increased gastric acid secretion and reduction in mucous production and mucosal blood flow. These effects and the acidic nature of the drug itself all increase risk of ulcer formation.

In the kidneys, prostaglandins maintain afferent arteriolar dilatation, regulating renal blood flow and glomerular filtration rate. They also have a role in the control of renin release and maintenance of water balance. NSAID inhibition of prostaglandin synthesis will result in reduction of renal blood flow and disrupt normal renal function and homeostatic mechanisms. Constriction of renal arterioles may result in renal papillary necrosis. These effects may be more evident in animals that are dehydrated or volume depleted.

Kinetics and metabolism

Diclofenac would appear to be readily absorbed in dogs as onset of clinical effects is usually within 2–3 hours of ingestion.

Clinical effects

The initial clinical effects following acute exposures usually occur within 3 hours. With more prolonged dosing, effects may be delayed for 4 days or more.

Clinical effects include persistent vomiting, haematemesis, diarrhoea, melena, abdominal tenderness and anorexia. Mucous membranes may be pale or congested. Weakness, ataxia, incoordination, lethargy, collapse, dehydration, depression and drowsiness are sometimes noted.

Dyspnoea, hyperventilation, tachycardia, vocalising, agitation, hyperactivity, hyperaesthesia, tremors, twitching or convulsions have been reported following ingestion of other similar drugs and could be anticipated. There is a risk of perforation of the gut.

From 12–24 hours post-dose onwards, evidence of severe gastrointestinal irritation and renal impairment may occur. There may be protracted vomiting, pyrexia, anorexia, polyuria, polydipsia, dehydration and collapse.

Renal impairment or failure should be anticipated if large doses (greater than 150–200 mg/kg body weight) have been ingested. This would be characterised by oliguria, azotemia, and elevated creatinine and BUN. Renal failure can theoretically occur and may be delayed. Hypotensive or dehydrated animals are potentially at greater risk from renal effects, as are those with pre-existing renal impairment.

Post-mortem findings

Evidence of gastrointestinal congestion and/or haemorrhage, gastric ulceration or perforation and renal tubule papillary necrosis would be anticipated.

Treatment

Treatment is advocated if a dose of 10 mg/kg body weight has been exceeded (5 mg/kg body weight in animals who are dehydrated, hypotensive or have pre-existing renal insufficiency).

If within 3 hours of ingestion, induce vomiting or perform gastric lavage and then administer adsorbents.

Emetics:

(a)	Apomorphine	Dose:	0.05 mg/kg body weight i.v. or i.m.; 0.1 mg/kg body weight s.c.
(b)	Xylazine	Dose:	0.2 mg/kg body weight i.v.; 0.5–1 mg/kg body weight i.m. or s.c.
(c)	Ipecacuanha	Dose:	1–2 ml/kg body weight (maximum 20 ml) orally
(d)	Soda crystal.		

Adsorbents:

(a)	Activated charcoal	Dose:	2g/kg body weight orally
(b)	BCK granules®	Dose:	6–18 g orally two or three times daily.

If there is severe or persistent vomiting then anti-emetics should be administered. If adsorbents have been administered this may reduce efficacy of orally administered anti-emetics. In such cases, parenteral administration is preferable. Either metoclopramide or acepromazine may be used; the latter has a longer duration of action.

(a)	Metoclopramide	Dose:	0.5–1 mg/kg body weight orally, s.c. or i.m. every 6–8 hours; 1–2 mg/kg body weight per day by slow i.v. infusion
(b)	Acepromazine	Dose:	0.03–0.1 mg/kg body weight i.v., i.m., or s.c. (use lower dose if giving i.v.); 1–3 mg/kg body weight orally.

Gastric effects

In *all* cases where treatment has been necessary the animals should be administered ulcer-healing or ulcer-preventing drugs.

The H_2-receptor blocking drugs cimetidine, ranitidine and famotidine reduce gastric acid and pepsin secretions, reducing the risk of ulcer formation and allowing ulcers to heal. Omeprazole inhibits the proton pump responsible for gastric acid production by the parietal cells. It is more potent and has a longer duration of action (greater than 24 hours) than the three aforementioned H$_2$-receptor blockers and its use should be reserved for animals who are not responding to other therapies.

Sucralfate is an ulcer-coating agent that binds to proteins at an ulcer site, protecting it from further gastric acid and pepsin attack.

Misoprostol is a synthetic prostaglandin analogue that in effect replaces the prostaglandins whose production is inhibited by diclofenac. Administration shortly after diclofenac sodium ingestion will therefore ensure continued control of gastric acid secretion and increased mucous production, thereby preventing ulcer formation. Its use is contra-indicated in animals who have already developed ulcers following NSAID ingestion.

Note: Some preparations present diclofenac sodium in combination with misoprostol.

Suggested regimen

The following treatment protocol is recommended for a 14-day period:

Either

Cimetidine   Dose: 5–10 mg/kg body weight i.v., i.m. or
                                   orally every 6–8 hours.

Notes

1. If adsorbents have been administered then parenteral routes should be employed in the initial stages.
2. If i.v. route is to be used then administer by slow i.v. injection over 30 minutes to reduce risk of hypotension and arrhythmias.
3. If metoclopramide has been used or sucralfate is to be used then a period of 2 hours should elapse before cimetidine is administered.
4. Adverse effect – cimetidine blocks liver microsomal enzymes and therefore hepatic drug metabolism.

Or

Ranitidine   Dose: 0.5–4 mg/kg body weight i.v., s.c. or
                                   orally every 12 hours.

Notes

1. If adsorbents have been administered then parenteral routes should be employed in the initial stages.
2. If metoclopramide has been used or sucralfate is to be used then a period of 2 hours should elapse before ranitidine is administered.

Or

Famotidine   Dose: 500 μg/kg body weight orally every
                                   12 hours.

Notes

1. Where adsorbents have been administered, a period of 2 hours should elapse before famotidine is administered, to minimise charcoal binding to drug.
2. If sucralfate is to be used then a period of 2 hours should elapse before famotidine is administered.

Where ingestion was recent and >10 mg/kg body weight of diclofenac sodium may have been ingested, also give

Misoprostol   Dose: 1–5 µg/kg body weight orally every 6–8 hours for 24 hours.

Notes

1. If a combination product that contains misoprostol was ingested then administration is not indicated.
2. Where adsorbents have been administered, a period of 2 hours should elapse before misoprostol is administered, to minimise charcoal binding to drug.
3. If ulceration is already suspected or confirmed, misoprostol should not be given and sucralfate given instead.
4. Adverse effects – misoprostol may cause vomiting, diarrhoea and abdominal tenderness and abortions in pregnant animals.

Where >10 mg/kg body weight diclofenac sodium may have been ingested and ulceration is either suspected or confirmed, give:

Sucralfate   Dose: in dogs <20 kg body weight 500 mg/dog orally every 6–8 hours; in dogs >20 kg body weight 1 g/dog orally every 6–8 hours.

Notes

1. Where adsorbents have been administered, a period of 2 hours should elapse before sucralfate is administered to minimise charcoal binding to drug.
2. If cimetidine, ranitidine or famotidine are to be used then sucralfate should be given 2 hours beforehand as it requires an acid environment for maximum efficacy.
3. Ideally, sucralfate should be administered on an empty stomach, at least 1 hour prior to food.

If the animal does not respond to the above therapies then administration of omeprazole may be considered. The recommended dose is 0.5–1.5 mg/kg body weight orally every 24 hours.

Other care

Management is otherwise largely symptomatic and supportive. Ensure adequate hydration and good urine output. In some cases, dopamine may be necessary to increase renal perfusion and to minimise renal insufficiency (dose: 1–3 µg/kg body weight per minute as constant i.v. infusion).

If possible, blood gases and electrolytes should be checked and corrected, especially if there is evidence of renal dysfunction and/or oliguria. Bicarbonate should be given to correct acidosis if present. *Caution* – dopamine precipitates in bicarbonate solutions, so these fluids should not be administered together. If the animal is hyperkalaemic then this should be corrected using dextrose (dose: 20% solution given 1 ml/kg body weight i.v.) together with insulin if available (dose: 0.5 units/kg body weight).

Diazepam may be given if there is any convulsant activity (dose: 0.5 mg/kg body weight i.v. repeated every 10 minutes up to three times if needed).

Bland diets are recommended.

Investigative

Blood levels are not helpful in management, except as confirmation of ingestion. Interpretation of levels is difficult and case management is better based on clinical condition of the animal. In any event, such analysis is not routinely offered by many laboratories.

In severe cases radiography, or gastroscopy may be employed to assess gastric mucosal damage.

References and further reading

VPIS (London) past cases up to 97/66762.

Giannoukas AD *et al.* (1996). Protection of the gastroduodenal mucosa from the effects of diclofenac sodium: role of highly selective vagotomy and misoprostol. *World Journal of Surgery* **20(4)**, 501–505.

Jones RD *et al.* (1992). Non-steroidal anti-inflammatory drug toxicosis in dogs and cats: 240 cases. *Journal of the American Veterinary Medical Association* **201(3)**, 475–478.

Kore AM (1990). Toxicology of non-steroidal anti-inflammatory drugs. *Veterinary Clinics of North America: Small Animal Practice* **20**, 419–429.

Kore AM (1997). Over-the-counter analgesic drug toxicoses in small animals. *Veterinary Medicine* **92(2)**, 158–165.

Lascelles D and Balmer T (1997). Are all NSAIDs the same? *Veterinary Times* **24(4)**, 34–37.

Vollmar AM (1993). Clinico-toxicologic aspects of non-steroidal anti-inflammatory agents in the dog and cat. *Tierarztliche Praxis* **21(2)**, 149–152.

Dieffenbachia

The plant

Common names include: Leopard Lily, Dumb Cane and Mother-in-Law's Tongue. These plants belong to the Araliaceae family.

Common as houseplants, they may grow up to 2 m in height. They bear large, variegated leaves of 10–25 cm length, ranging in colour from dark green to pale green or yellow and flower occasionally. Varieties commonly found in the UK do not usually produce fruits.

Occurrence of poisoning incidences

Since the launch of the VPIS, the centre in London has received a small number of enquiries regarding ingestion of dieffenbachia by domestic pets. The majority of these enquiries involve dogs. Most have displayed mild to moderate clinical effects only and all have made a full recovery.

Mechanism of toxicity

The plant contains high concentrations of calcium oxalate needles and oxalic acid, both of which are very irritant to mucous membranes and may also result in histamine release. Other plants from this family also contain proteolytic enzymes, which may further exacerbate the irritant effects.

Clinical effects

Onset of clinical effects in small animals is usually within 4 hours.

Common effects include hypersalivation, vomiting, severe diarrhoea, anorexia and often evidence of severe irritation of buccal mucous membranes. Some animals have exhibited marked abdominal tenderness, colic and depression.

Treatment

Gastric decontamination is unnecessary.

Management is supportive, allowing the animals access to plenty of fluid. For large ingestions, evaluation of oral mucosa and tongue for signs of severe swelling is recommended.

Reference

VPIS (London) past case up to 97/75144.

Ethylene glycol

Type of product

Ethylene glycol is most commonly encountered in antifreeze, screenwash or, more rarely, de-icers. Most antifreezes available contain ethylene glycol or methanol.

Presentation

Antifreeze is available as a liquid to be added to water in engine radiators to prevent freezing and improve hot-weather performance, the usual final dilution being 1:3 or 1:4.

It is apparently sweet-tasting and palatable and dogs, in particular, appear to like to drink it.

Occurrence of poisoning incidence

Since 1992, the VPIS has received a small number of enquiries every year regarding the ingestion of ethylene glycol-containing products by companion animals. The majority of these cases involve dogs. A few fatal cases are reported. In the most severe case, a 3-year-old St Bernard drank from a bucket of liquid drained from a car radiator. By 36 hours the dog had ataxia, lethargy, continuous vomiting and renal failure. The dog was euthanased after 7 days of supportive care (VPISLn case 84/35372). Ethylene glycol poisoning is more commonly reported in the winter months.

Toxicity

According to the literature:

- The quoted lethal dose of ethylene glycol for dogs is 6.6 ml/kg body weight.
- In 35 cases of ingestion of ethylene glycol in dogs the mortality rate was 70.4% (Rowland, 1987).

Mechanism of toxicity

The major toxic agent in ethylene glycol poisoning is not the parent compound but the metabolites produced by the action of alcohol dehydrogenase on the parent compound. Alcohol dehydrogenase converts ethylene glycol to glycoaldehyde. This is then metabolised to glycolic acid, which appears to be the principal cause of the acidosis. One of the metabolites of glycolic acid is oxalate, which causes renal damage, and hypocalcaemia by binding to calcium to form calcium oxalate, crystals of which appear in the urine. The aldehydes (glycoaldehyde, glycolic acid and glyoxylate) may inhibit oxidative phosphorylation and respiration. Glycolic acid is metabolised to glycine, which is metabolised to hippurate.

Kinetics

Ethylene glycol is quickly absorbed from the gastrointestinal tract.

Clinical effects
Stage 1 (30 minutes–12 hours)

Central nervous system signs including vomiting, ataxia, tachycardia, weakness and convulsions; also polydipsia, polyuria, dehydration, tachypnoea, acidosis, hypothermia.

Stage 2 (12–24 hours)

Cardiopulmonary signs including tachypnoea, tachycardia, pulmonary oedema, hyperaemia and congestion. There may be transient recovery followed by anorexia, severe depression, coma and convulsions.

Stage 3 (24–72 hours)

Renal system signs including oliguria, azotaemia and/or uraemia, vomiting, anorexia and severe depression. Renal failure indicates a poor prognosis.

Recovery may take 3–4 weeks; however, in some cases there may be irreversible renal tubular damage.

The longer the delay before initiation of treatment, the less favourable the prognosis. Animals that have improving clinical signs after 10–16 hours of treatment have a favourable prognosis. However, in most cases unless the ingestion was witnessed, animals usually present in the third stage of poisoning and in these animals the prognosis is poor.

Laboratory findings

(a) Increased osmolality (normal 280–310 mOsm/kg): an osmolality raised by as much as 60 mOsm/kg is typical of ethylene glycol poisoning.
(b) Increased anion gap (normal 10–12 mEq/L): an anion gap >40–50 mEq/L is typical of ethylene glycol poisoning.
(c) Acidosis: pH usually <7.3, urine pH usually <6.5.
(d) Renal damage: raised urea and creatinine, low urine specific gravity, calcium oxalate crystals (may appear within 5 hours of ingestion), proteinuria, glucosuria, haematuria and albuminuria. Calcium oxalate crystals are light yellow, arranged in rosettes, sheaves or prisms and are birefringent (transmit light unequally in different directions) in polarised light.
(e) Hyperglycaemia, hypocalcaemia, hyperphosphataemia, hyperkalaemia.

(f) Neutrophil leucocytosis, eosinopaenia (Johnson *et al.*, 1979).
(g) Raised ethylene glycol concentrations in blood and urine.
(h) Hippurate and oxalate detected in urine.

Post-mortem findings

(a) Gastrointestinal tract: gastric mucosa haemorrhagic and hyperaemic.
(b) Pulmonary hyperaemia and oedema.
(c) Kidney: pale, swollen with grey or yellow streaks, particularly near the corticomedullary junction. Oxalate crystals are usually present in the kidney. In animals that survive, regenerating renal tubules are dilated and lined with flattened tubular epithelium.

Diagnosis

Ethylene glycol poisoning may be mistaken for head trauma, encephalitis, acute gastroenteritis, pancreatitis, ketoacidotic diabetes mellitus and acute renal failure from other causes. Diagnosis is based on history, clinical signs and laboratory data. Abdominal palpation may be painful due to renal oedema. Ethylene glycol poisoning should be suspected in any animal with the following:

(a) acute onset of signs;
(b) raised urea, creatinine and other nitrogenous compounds in the blood (azotaemia or uraemia);
(c) low or fixed urine specific gravity (Grauer and Thrall, 1982).

Treatment

Therapy for ethylene glycol is principally aimed at blocking the action of alcohol dehydrogenase to prevent the formation of the toxic metabolites. This is achieved by the administration of the preferred substrate, ethanol, which allows renal excretion of the unmetabolised parent compound. In untreated dogs the half-life of ethylene glycol was about 6 hours, but this was doubled in dogs treated with ethanol. 4-Methylpyrazole (4-MP, fomepizole) a direct inhibitor of alcohol dehydrogenase, has been suggested as an alternative therapy to ethanol on the grounds of a lack of adverse effects and slower elimination. Clinical reports suggest that 4-MP is successful in treating ethylene glycol intoxication in dogs. It is currently undergoing clinical trials in the USA and Europe for the treatment of ethylene glycol poisoning in humans.

If within 2 hours of ingestion, induce vomiting or perform gastric lavage. Adsorbents are not useful.

Emetics:

(a) Apomorphine	Dose:	0.05 mg/kg body weight i.v. or i.m.; 0.1 mg/kg body weight s.c.
(b) Xylazine	Dose:	0.2 mg/kg body weight i.v.; 0.5–1 mg/kg body weight i.m. or s.c.

Dogs | 129

(c) Ipecacuanha   Dose: 1–2 ml/kg body weight (maximum
                                         20 ml) orally

(d) Soda crystal.

Monitor pH and renal function. Correct acidosis with sodium bicarbonate (see below). Fluids should be given to ensure adequate hydration and a good urine output. Central venous pressure and renal output should be monitored in dogs with renal dysfunction because of the risk of fluid overload and subsequent pulmonary oedema. Mannitol can be used in a well-hydrated animal to produce an osmotic diuresis and reduce renal oedema.

Dose: 0.25–0.5 g/kg body weight i.v. over 5–10 minutes.

Peritoneal dialysis is recommended in acidotic dogs with oliguria.

Antidotal therapy

Ethanol is a specific antidote (see above for mechanism) and should be given in any symptomatic case presenting within 24 hours; however, it is probably most effective if given within 12 hours of ingestion. (Note: There is no point in giving ethanol to block metabolism if the ethylene glycol has been metabolised.) Cases often present late, by which time antidotal therapy is no longer of use. Management is supportive. Ethanol should not be given to dogs with renal failure.

Ethanol regimen

Either: 5.5 ml/kg body weight 20% ethanol in saline i.v. every 4 hours for five doses then every 6 hours for four doses;

or: a loading dose of 1.4 ml/kg body weight of 20% ethanol i.v. over 15 minutes, followed by an i.v. infusion of 0.62 ml/kg body weight/hour for 48–56 hours.

Note: in human poisoning cases, once diagnosis has been confirmed by a laboratory, the ethanol given as treatment is given either orally or intravenously. In these cases, the recommended doses for 5% and 10% ethanol solutions are identical whatever the route of administration. Therefore, if ethanol in a form suitable for injection is not readily available, an equivalent dosing to the above, suitably diluted, could be given orally (ideally by tube direct into the stomach) as an interim measure, e.g. 0.5–0.7 ml/kg body weight per hour of a 40% spirit suitably diluted.

Use of ethanol-containing preparations such as methylated spirits or surgical spirits is not recommended as these preparations both contain small quantities (about 5%) of methanol.

4-MP regimen (if available)

Loading dose: 20 mg/kg body weight as a 5% solution i.v., then 15 mg/kg body weight at 12 and 24 hours, followed by 5 mg/kg at 36 hours. If ethylene glycol is still detected in the blood then 5 mg/kg should be given every 12 hours.

Bicarbonate regimen

The aim is to keep the urine pH at about 7.5–8.0.

(a) With known laboratory analyses:

$$\text{mmol (mEq) of bicarbonate required} = \frac{\text{base deficit} \times 0.5 \times \text{body weight (kg)}}{2}$$

Give slowly over 3–4 hours i.v. Recheck blood gases and assess the clinical status of the animal.

(b) If blood gases are not available:

give 0.5–1 mmol/kg body weight i.v. slowly over 30 minutes.

Dogs may eat and drink during treatment, although those on ethanol therapy may have CNS depression and may therefore require parenteral or tube feeding.

Calculations

anion gap = $(Na^+ + K^+) - (HCO_3^{\ -} + Cl^-)$

osmolar gap = measured osmolality − calculated osmolality

calculated osmolality (mOsmol/kg H_2O) =

$$\frac{(1.86 \times [\text{Na in mmol/L}]) + (\text{urea in mmol/L}) + (\text{glucose in mmol/L})}{0.93}$$

References

VPIS (London) past cases up to 97/186001.

Beckett SD and Shields RP (1971). Treatment of acute ethylene glycol (antifreeze) toxicosis in dogs. *Journal of the American Veterinary Association* **158(4)**, 472–476.

Dial SM, Thrall MAH and Hamar DW (1989). 4-Methylpyrazole as treatment for naturally acquired ethylene glycol intoxication in dogs. *Journal of the American Veterinary Association* **195(1)**, 73–76.

Dial SM, Thrall MAH and Hamar DW (1994). Efficacy of 4-methylpyrazole for treatment of ethylene glycol intoxication in dogs. *American Journal of Veterinary Research* **55(12)**, 1762–1770.

Fox LE *et al.* (1987). Reversal of ethylene glycol-induced nephrotoxicosis in a dog. *Journal of the American Veterinary Association* **191(11)**, 1433–1435.

Grauer GF and Thrall MA (1982). Ethylene glycol (antifreeze) poisoning in the dogs and cat. *Journal of the American Animal Hospital Association* **18**, 492–497.

Herd P (1992). Poison – ethylene glycol. *In Practice* **14(6)**, 298–299.

Johnson SE *et al.* (1979). Current status of ethylene glycol toxicity in dogs – a review. *Minnesota Veterinarian* **2**, 32–43.

Proudfoot AT (1993). *Acute Poisoning. Diagnosis and Management* (second edition). Oxford: Butterworth-Heinemann, pp. 120–123.

Rowland J (1987). Incidence of ethylene glycol intoxication in dogs and cats seen at Colorado State University Veterinary Teaching Hospital. *Veterinary and Human Toxicology* **29(1)**, 41–44.

Tarr BD *et al.* (1985). Low-dose ethanol in the treatment of ethylene glycol poisoning. *Journal of Veterinary Pharmacology and Therapy* **8**, 254–262.

Thrall MA, Grauer GF and Mero KN (1984). Clinicopathologic findings in dogs and cats with ethylene glycol intoxication. *Journal of the American Veterinary Association* **184(1)**, 37–41.

Fertilisers

Type of product

Fertilisers are used as for gardening and agricultural purposes.

Presentation

A variety of amateur and professional products are available. Both indoor and outdoor domestic fertilisers tend to be 'NPK' based; that is, the primary constituents are nitrogen, phosphorous and potassium. To these may be added trace elements such as iron chelate or manganese. Houseplant fertilisers are usually liquid preparations, diluted before use, although tablets and sticks are also available. Outdoor fertilisers may be powder, granules or liquid, again usually diluted. Phosphorus may be in the form of animal bone (bone meal) or phosphorous pentoxide.

Note: Some fertilisers contain a high concentration of iron (usually iron sulphate), which may cause iron poisoning – see iron and iron salts chapter. Lawn fertilisers may also contain small quantities of herbicides and/or fungicides.

Occurrence of poisoning incidences

Since the launch of the VPIS, the centre in London has received up to at least 25 enquiries per year regarding ingestion of fertiliser products by animals. In 1997, 93 enquiries of this nature were received, accounting for 2.8% of the total enquiries. These enquires predominantly involve dogs.

Toxicity

Fertilisers are generally of low toxicity. In most cases, only gastrointestinal irritation is reported.

According to the literature:

- Dogs fed 10 mg/kg of a herbicide/fertiliser mixture did not exhibit clinical signs of toxicity. The doses of the constituents given in mg/kg body weight were urea 623, phosphorous pentoxide 24, potassium oxide 66, 2,4-D 6.51, MCPP 3.26, dicamba 0.55 and bensulide 60.93. The dosing regimen used was equivalent to ingestion of 0.06 m^2 lawn/kg body weight, with the fertiliser mixture applied at the recommended application rate. This exceeds the quantity of grass that animals typically ingest, which is about 5–10 g.

In the experience of VPISLn:

- Over 150 cases are on file, where follow-up data are available. In over 55% of these cases the animals were asymptomatic.
- One fatal case is documented. The dog developed severe gastro-intestinal discomfort, with blood-stained diarrhoea. It is possible that the preparation ingested contained ferrous sulphate (VPISLn case 94/136580).

Mechanism of toxicity

It is considered that most clinical effects following ingestion of fertilisers result from the irritant nature of the constituents.

Clinical effects

Onset of effects is usually between 2–10 hours post-ingestion. Duration of gastrointestinal effects has been 12 hours in some past VPISLn cases.

Vomiting, diarrhoea, salivation, polydipsia, lethargy and abdominal tenderness are the most likely effects.

Rarely reported effects include shivering, transient hindleg stiffness, swelling of the muzzle, urticarial rash formation and itching. Two dogs developed altered behaviour (hiding and lying in the rain), which was attributed to the ingestion.

Treatment

Gastric emptying and adsorbents are unlikely to be required.

Treatment is symptomatic and supportive, particularly ensuring adequate hydration. An anti-emetic may be used if there is excessive vomiting. Either metoclopramide or acepromazine may be used; the latter has a longer duration of action.

(a) Metoclopramide	Dose:	0.5–1 mg/kg body weight orally, s.c. or i.m. every 6–8 hours; 1–2 mg/kg body weight per day by slow i.v. infusion
(b) Acepromazine	Dose:	0.03–0.1 mg/kg body weight i.v., i.m., or s.c. (use lower dose if giving i.v.); 1–3 mg/kg body weight orally.

References and further reading

VPIS (London) past cases up to 96/149473.

Yeary RA (1984). Oral intubation of dogs with combinations of fertilizer, herbicide and insecticide chemicals commonly used on lawns. *American Journal of Veterinary Research* **45(2)**, 288–290.

Glyphosate

Type of product

Glyphosate is a broad-spectrum post-emergence herbicide. It is an organophosphate herbicide with *no* anticholinesterase activity, widely used because it is of low toxicity, lacks residual soil activity, does not bioaccumulate and is biodegradable.

Presentation

Amateur and professional products are available. Glyphosate is primarily used in the isopropylamine salt and is available in liquid formulations. These are of variable strengths, but most of those commonly available contain between 120 and 500 g/L of glyphosate, i.e. 12–50% w/v.

Occurrence of poisoning incidences

Since the launch of the VPIS, the centre in London has received up to 45 enquiries per annum regarding animals who have poisoning attributed to glyphosate-containing products. Over 95% of these cases involve dogs. Poisoning has usually been attributed to ingestion of grass and vegetation recently treated with a glyphosate-based herbicide. A number of fatal cases have occurred, five in dogs and three in cats.

Toxicity

The toxicity has not been distinguished from that of the formulated products. A surfactant, polyoxyethylene amine (POEA), present in many liquid preparations, may be responsible for some of the effects, particularly with the professional products. The surfactant aids adsorption of the herbicide onto plants. Some products contain up to 15% surfactant.

According to the literature:

- 150 ppm is the expected concentration in grass from recommended application rate.
- 2000 ppm is the no-effect dietary concentration in long-term feeding trials in dogs.
- Beagles fed 0–500 mg/kg/day (in gelatine capsules) for approximately 1 year showed no clinical signs of toxicity.
- There is limited information on dogs but the LD_{50} in other animals is high: mice >10 000 mg/kg, rats >5000 mg/kg, rabbits 3800 mg/kg, goats >3500 mg/kg.
- There is limited information on the toxicity of POEA, but in rats the LD_{50} is 1280–1300 mg/kg, which is about one-third that of glyphosate.

In the experience of VPISLn:

- The cases reported often involve dogs eating recently treated vegetation in parks or gardens. Over 150 canine cases have been reported to the VPISLn, of which approximately 40% remained asymptomatic. Approximately 45% have mild to moderate effects and the remainder would be classified as serious. Five fatal cases in dogs have been reported.

In common with the findings of a French survey of enquiries to a veterinary poisons information centre, the enquiries about glyphosate products occur predominantly in spring and early summer. This correlates with the agricultural use of glyphosate.

- A 9-year-old Labrador was presented with spasms, panting, shaking, hind-leg ataxia and muscle spasms after ingestion of a glyphosate-containing herbicide. The animal was treated with i.v. diazepam, atropine and steroids and made a slow recovery (VPISLn case 93/80395).
- A 40 kg German Shepherd dog was admitted with ataxia, disorientation and convulsions after ingestion of a herbicide preparation. The animal was treated symptomatically but deteriorated rapidly and was euthanased (VPISLn case 94/40272).
- A 6-year-old Airedale was presented with melena, pale mucous membranes, icterus, pyrexia and haematuria after ingestion of herbicide. The animal was given vitamin K_1, steroids, antibiotics and plasma expanders, but died (VPISLn case 95/116804).
- A 22 kg mongrel ate herbicide-treated grass. It presented with diarrhoea, inappetence, and icterus. Laparotomy revealed a fibrosed and cirrhotic liver. The animal was euthanased (VPISLn case 96/46988).

Mechanism of toxicity

The toxic mechanisms of glyphosate have not been determined. It may uncouple oxidative phosphorylation. POEA is irritant.

Kinetics and metabolism

There is limited information on kinetics of glyphosate in dogs. In laboratory animals (rats and rabbits), absorption from the gastrointestinal tract is poor and retention of glyphosate in tissues is low. The majority of absorbed glyphosate is excreted unchanged in the urine or faeces.

Clinical effects

Onset of clinical effects is usually between 30 minutes and 2 hours. Recovery usually occurs over 1–2 days.

Salivation, vomiting, diarrhoea, irritation and swelling of lips are common early features. Tachycardia, and excitability are often present in the early stages, with the animals subsequently becoming ataxic, depressed and bradycardic. Inappetence, pharyngitis, pyrexia, twitching, shaking and dilated pupils are noted occasionally. Rarely, jaundice, hepatic damage and haematuria have been reported. Eye and skin irritation are also possible.

Tachypnoea occurs in glyphosate poisoning in other animals but does not appear to be a feature of glyphosate toxicity in dogs.

In severe cases collapse, severe bradycardia and convulsions may occur.

Post-mortem findings

No dog data are available in the literature. Pulmonary hyperaemia is the main feature in rats and mice.

Treatment

If within 2 hours of ingestion, induce vomiting or perform gastric lavage, and then administer adsorbents.

Emetics:

(a) Apomorphine	Dose:	0.05 mg/kg body weight i.v. or i.m.; 0.1 mg/kg body weight s.c.
(b) Xylazine	Dose:	0.2 mg/kg body weight i.v.; 0.5–1 mg/kg body weight i.m. or s.c.
(c) Ipecacuanha	Dose:	1–2 ml/kg body weight (maximum 20 ml) orally
(d) Soda crystal.		

Adsorbents:

(a) Activated charcoal	Dose:	2 g/kg body weight orally
(b) BCK granules®	Dose:	6–18 g orally two or three times daily.

If there is severe or persistent vomiting then anti-emetics should be administered. If adsorbents have been administered this may reduce efficacy of orally administered anti-emetics. In such cases, parenteral administration is preferable. Either metoclopramide or acepromazine may be used; the latter has a longer duration of action.

(a) Metoclopramide	Dose:	0.5–1 mg/kg body weight orally, s.c. or i.m. every 6–8 hours; 1–2 mg/kg body weight per day by slow i.v. infusion
(b) Acepromazine	Dose:	0.03–0.1 mg/kg body weight i.v., i.m., or s.c. (use lower dose if giving i.v.); 1–3 mg/kg body weight orally.

If there is a risk of dermal exposure the animal should be thoroughly washed. Treatment thereafter is largely supportive. Intravenous fluid support should be given to maintain hydration if required. Liver function tests should be considered if the animal displays serious clinical effects.

References and further reading

VPIS (London) cases up to 97/95765.

Burgat V *et al.* (1998). Glyphosate toxicosis in domestic animals: a survey from the data of the Centre National d'Informations Toxicologiques Vétérinaires (CNITV). *Veterinary and Human Toxicology* **40(6)**, 363–368.

Smith EA and Oehme FW (1992). The biological activity of glyphosate to plants and animals: a literature review. *Veterinary and Human Toxicology* **34(6)**, 531–543.

Holly / *Ilex aquifolium*

The plant

Common name: Holly. The plant belongs to the Aquifolianeae family.

This is a commonly encountered evergreen shrub with characteristic glossy, leathery, dark green leaves with spiky margins. The plant flowers in late spring to early summer with yellow–green or pinkish blooms. The female plants bear fruits, which remain on the plant through out the winter. The rounded fleshy berries are usually bright red, sometimes yellow or black, and grow in clusters.

Occurrence of poisoning incidences

Since the launch of the VPIS, the centre in London has received a small number of enquiries each year regarding ingestion of holly leaves and/or berries. These cases have largely involved dogs. Cases with clinical effects are rare.

Toxicity

The plant is considered by the VPIS to be of low toxicity.

According to the literature:

● Reportedly, 20 berries may cause fatality in a large dog. This appears unsubstantiated by case data.

Mechanism of toxicity

Potentially, all parts of the plant are toxic. The leaves and berries contain saponins such as ilicin, ilexanthin and ilicic acid, which have local irritant effects on mucous membranes. The leaves, berries and stems also contain cyanogenic glycosides. Presence of triterpenes and a compound with digitalis-type activity has also been documented.

Clinical effects

Clinical effects are rare, but the spiny nature of the leaves presumably renders then unattractive for consumption.

Effects would be anticipated within 2–3 hours. Ingestion may result in vomiting (which may be severe or protracted), diarrhoea and salivation. Inappetence and depression have been described in a few past VPIS cases.

Treatment

Gastric decontamination using gastric lavage, emesis or adsorbents is not necessary as the berries are of low toxicity and vomiting usually occurs spontaneously.

Use of metoclopramide may be considered if vomiting is severe. Dose: 0.5–1 mg/kg body weight orally, s.c. or i.m. every 6–8 hours; 1–2 mg/kg body weight per day by slow i.v. infusion.

Management should otherwise be supportive, particularly ensuring that the animal is well hydrated.

References and further reading

VPIS (London) past cases up to 96/3398.

Willems M (1989). Quantitative determination and distribution of a cyanogenic glycoside in Ilex aquifolium. *Planta Medica* **55**, 195.

Waud RA (1932). A digitalis-like action of extracts made from holly. *Journal of Pharmacology and Experimental Therapeutics* **45**, 279.

Honeysuckle / *Lonicera* species

The plant

Common species are: *Lonicera peridymenum* (Common honeysuckle, woodbine), *Lonicera xylosteum* (Fly honeysuckle) and *Lonicera caprifolium* (Perfoliate honeysuckle)

There are numerous different species of honeysuckle and many cultivars and hybrids. Honeysuckle is a many-branched spreading shrub or a woody climber, with stems up to 6 m long. It is a member of the Caprifoliaceae family. The leaves are variable in shape but often dark green with a pale green underside. The flowers appear from May to late September; in the Common honeysuckle they are yellowish-white with a purplish tinge.

The berries vary in colour but the common species have bright red round berries approximately 8–9 mm in diameter. These occur in dense clusters of between 5 and 15. Inside the berries are six oval, yellow seeds. The flesh is juicy and sometimes the berries are sticky and covered in dust, which dulls their appearance. The berries ripen from August to September.

Occurrence of poisoning incidences

Since the launch of the VPIS, the centre in London has received a small number of enquiries each year regarding ingestion of honeysuckle. All these cases have involved dogs. Usually berries have been consumed. Clinical effects are usually mild and no fatal cases have been reported.

Toxicity

The plant is generally considered of low toxicity. Cases reported to the VPISLn have usually displayed mild gastrointestinal effects only.

Mechanism of toxicity

Honeysuckle fruits contain valerianic acid and xylostein, which are irritant.

Clinical effects

Onset of effects is usually within 2 hours. The common effects are vomiting, diarrhoea (may be bloody), depression and lethargy. Convulsions were reported by the owner of one dog in a VPISLn case (93/81260).

Treatment

Gastric emptying is unnecessary and vomiting usually occur spontaneously. Ensure that the animal is adequately hydrated.

If there is severe or persistent vomiting, metoclopramide may be given. Dose: 0.5–1 mg/kg body weight orally, s.c. or i.m. every 6–8 hours; 1–2 mg/kg body weight per day by slow i.v. infusion.

Reference

VPIS (London) past cases up to 96/162522.

Horse chestnut / *Aesculus hippocastanum*

The plant

Common names are: Horse chestnut or 'conker'. The plants belong to the Hippocastanaceae family.

Aesculus hippocastanum is a large deciduous tree up to 25 m high, found in parks and urban areas. The large, oval buds are covered with red-brown sticky bud scales. The leaves consist of between five and seven leaflets, each up to 15 cm long. The clusters of white, pink or deep red flowers appear from April to June. The fruits are large spiny, green to yellow or brown capsules, which contain one or more shiny brown seeds (the conkers), which ripen from August to October.

Occurrence of poisoning incidences

Since 1993, the VPIS London centre has received between five and 15 enquiries per annum regarding ingestion of horse chestnuts by dogs. Most of these cases are reported in the autumn, when the fruits ripen. All but one case reported have displayed clinical effects. Two fatal cases are reported.

Toxicity

In the experience of the VPISLn:

- A 10 kg, 14-month-old, cross-bred dog consumed at least eight horse chestnuts. The dog collapsed, vomited profusely, became dehydrated and went into toxic shock. The dog was rehydrated, given prednisolone, multivitamins, antibiotics and a gastrotomy performed to remove plant material from the gut. The animal returned 3 days later, after a possible repeat ingestion, but on this occasion died shortly after presentation (VPISLn case 96/154594).

Mechanism of toxicity

The poisonous principle is aesculin, a saponin glycoside (7-hydroxycoumarin-6-glucoside), though aesculin is sometimes used as a collective term for the saponins in this plant. Young leaves and flowers are considered to be the most toxic part of the plant. The bark contains the highest aesculin concentration, but this part is rarely eaten. Alkaloids may also be present. The seed (conker) contains a large amount of starch and 3–5% aesculin.

Clinical effects

Onset can occur within 1–6 hours, but in most cases it has been 2 days.

Effects include vomiting, diarrhoea, salivation, haematemesis, abdominal tenderness, polydipsia, anorexia and dehydration; also restlessness, ataxia, muscle tremor, rigidity, pyrexia, partial paralysis and obstruction of the gastrointestinal tract. In one fatal case reported to the VPIS, respiratory paralysis occurred.

Treatment

If within 2 hours of ingestion, induce vomiting or perform gastric lavage. Adsorbents are unlikely to be of any benefit and may exacerbate obstruction.

Emetics:

(a)	Apomorphine	Dose:	0.05 mg/kg body weight i.v. or i.m.; 0.1 mg/kg body weight s.c.
(b)	Xylazine	Dose:	0.2 mg/kg body weight i.v.; 0.5–1 mg/kg body weight i.m. or s.c.
(c)	Ipecacuanha	Dose:	1–2 ml/kg body weight (maximum 20 ml) orally
(d)	Soda crystal.		

Treatment is otherwise supportive, particularly ensuring that the animal does not become dehydrated.

If there is severe or persistent vomiting, metoclopramide may be given. Dose: 0.5–1 mg/kg body weight orally, s.c. or i.m. every 6–8 hours; 1–2 mg/kg body weight per day by slow i.v. infusion.

Laparotomy and surgical removal of impacted plant material may be required in dogs with obstruction. Ventilation may be required in dogs with severe respiratory distress.

Reference

VPIS (London) past cases up to 97/39819.

Hymenoptera

The insects

These insects are part of a group that includes bees, wasps, and hornets. They are characterised by the possession of two pairs of wings, one pair of antennae, three body segments and, in the females, stinging apparatus at the end of the abdomen.

The stinging apparatus varies from species to species. Bees have a barbed stinger with lancets that firmly attach to the skin of the victim during the attack. Stinging therefore results in the tearing off of the apparatus from the abdomen and the subsequent death of the insect. The reflex action of the stinger muscles may, however, continue to inject more venom into the victim. Wasps and hornets have unbarbed stingers and are therefore capable of inflicting multiple stings on their victims.

Occurrence of poisoning incidences

Since 1992, the VPIS London centre has received a small number of enquiries each year regarding bee, wasp and hornet stings in animals. To date, all of these have been in dogs. Several cases have involved multiple stings.

Toxicity

Hymenoptera stings may result in localised pain and swelling, and only very rarely cause severe toxicity. Severe anaphylactic reactions are reported to occur in animals sensitive to the insect venom, occasionally resulting in fatality. Deaths have occurred as a result of upper airway blockage through oedema caused by stings in the mouth or on the neck or head.

The venom of africanised honeybees (so-called killer bees), which are found in parts of the USA, is similar to that of domesticated honeybees. It is no more toxic or allergenic than that of domesticated honeybees. These bees, however, are more aggressive and the risk of multiple stings is greater.

In the experience of the VPISLn:

- A 1-year-old collie disturbed a beehive and received multiple stings. It howled constantly, vomited profusely, with the vomitus containing many insects. It became lethargic. Evidence of multiple stings was present inside the mouth. The animal developed severe haemolytic anaemia. The animal was managed supportively with corticosteroids, plasma expanders and intravenous fluid therapy and a blood transfusion. The clinical effects persisted for 6 days but the animal made a full recovery (VPISLn case 87/29396).

Mechanism of toxicity

The venom compositions are variable but most contain phospholipases, phosphatases and hyaluronidase components, together with histamine. The latter contributes to the pain and inflammatory response.

Clinical effects

In dogs, stings to the facial area are complicating, as their panting is a means of control of body temperature and the swelling that may occur following stings may impair thermoregulation.

Local reactions: normal reactions to a sting include immediate pain, redness, and inflammation. The animal may bark or yelp continuously. The area local to the site of the sting may become irritating and swollen. If the sting is on the tongue or in the mouth, the local swelling may potentially cause respiratory distress.

Toxic reactions: these normally occur with multiple stings. The clinical effects include local reactions as above, with vomiting, diarrhoea, hypotension, fever and very rarely transient drowsiness, convulsions, anaemia and renal failure being reported. Cardiovascular and respiratory collapse of rapid onset have also been reported.

Allergic reactions: in sensitised animals a single sting may produce serious, potentially fatal, anaphylactic reactions, usually within 30 minutes. Clinical effects include bronchospasm and collapse.

Treatment

Treatment of local reactions need only be supportive, with the use of antihistamines (e.g. chlorpheniramine) if deemed necessary. Steroids may be given for severe local swelling or if the sting is to the mouth or facial regions (e.g. beclomethasone, dexamethasone, methylprednisolone).

If the sting was from a bee, the stinger should be removed by flicking or scraping with a fingernail, piece of card or knife blade. The stinger should *not* be squeezed or pulled from the skin, since this may release more venom into the wound.

Toxic reactions will probably only require symptomatic and supportive care as for local reactions, with intravenous fluid support if required. Antibiotic cover is recommended.

Anaphylactic reactions require prompt treatment of bronchospasm and hypotension that may result. The use of adrenaline (1:1000 strength) is advocated for severe reactions. Dose: 20 μg/kg body weight i.v. (i.e. 0.02 ml/kg body weight of 0.1% solution (1:1000), diluted in 5–10 ml of normal saline).

Management is otherwise supportive. Where bees are involved, the stinger apparatus should be removed where possible. Where multiple stings have occurred, the animal should be checked for presence of anaemia.

References

VPIS (London) past cases up to 97/111980.

Antin IP (1963). Fatal anaphylactic reaction of dog to bee sting. *Journal of the American Veterinary Medical Association* **142**, 775.

Cowell A and Cowell R (1995). Management of bee and other hymenoptera stings. *Current Veterinary Therapy* **XII**, 226–228.

Ibuprofen

Type of product

Ibuprofen is a non-steroidal, anti-inflammatory, analgesic drug (NSAID).

Presentation

Ibuprofen is available in the UK both as a prescription medicine and as an 'over-the-counter' medication. It is sold under various brand names in both tablet and liquid suspension preparations. Topical preparations are also available.

The dose of ibuprofen in tablet preparations is variable but usually within a 200–800 mg range. Most 'over-the-counter' tablets contain 200 mg or 400 mg.

Some preparations may contain other drugs as well, e.g. codeine, pseudoephedrine. Liquid suspension preparations are commonly of 100 mg/5 ml strength. Topical preparations vary in strength but are commonly 5% w/v (i.e. 5 g/100 ml of gel).

Occurrence of poisoning incidences

Ibuprofen is the drug about which the VPIS is most frequently consulted. Since 1992, there has been a small increase in the percentage of the total enquiries that enquiries about ibuprofen represent (2.5% in 1992, rising to 4.3% in 1997). Over 95% of these cases involved ingestion by dogs.

Recommended dosage

In the UK the drug is supplied for use in humans only. There are *no* indications for the use of this drug in veterinary medicine. In dogs, particularly, its use is potentially very dangerous.

In the past, a dosage of 5 mg/kg body weight was advocated in the dog and used for anti-inflammatory and analgesic purposes without any damaging effects being reported, but prolonged daily doses of 8 mg/kg body weight have resulted in severe toxicity. Hence, the safety margin is a narrow one.

Toxicity

Dogs are particularly sensitive to the propionic acid group of NSAIDs (e.g. ibuprofen and flurbiprofen). In particular, they are prone to develop severe gastric ulceration and intestinal irritation.

A dose of 5 mg/kg body weight was the recommended therapeutic dose in dogs for analgesic and anti-inflammatory purposes. Such doses were not reported to result in toxicity.

Experimental doses of 8–16 mg/kg body weight given once daily for 30 days have been reported to cause mild gastrointestinal disturbances only, the severity increasing with dose. Post-mortem examination revealed gastric ulcers and erosion, and severe intestinal inflammation.

According to the literature:

- An acute dosing of 100 mg/kg body weight may cause moderate to severe toxicosis, with gastrointestinal effects predominant. With treatment full recovery is likely.
- Acute doses greater than 250 mg/kg body weight may cause renal impairment.
- A dose of 333 mg/kg body weight was reported to result in acute renal failure.
- Doses greater than 300 mg/kg body weight may result in fatality.
- German Shepherd dogs may be at greater risk.

In the experience of the VPISLn:

- Acute doses as low as 6 mg/kg body weight have caused gastro-intestinal effects (VPISLn case 95/150712).
- In some dogs, acute doses greater than 200 mg/kg body weight have been survived with treatment, and caused no apparent clinical effects (e.g. VPISLn cases 94/141798 and 96/139572).

Mechanism of toxicity

Ibuprofen competitively inhibits the cyclo-oxygenase step of prostaglandin synthesis. Such inhibition and subsequent reduction in levels of PGI_2 and PGE_2 can account for the major effects seen in poisoning cases.

In the gastrointestinal tract prostaglandins have a cytoprotective function, as they control production of gastric acid, stimulate secretion of mucous and bicarbonate by the gastric epithelium and maintain mucosal blood flow by causing vasodilatation. Deficiency will result in increased gastric acid secretion and reduction in mucous production and mucosal blood flow. These effects and the acidic nature of the drug itself all increase risk of ulcer formation.

In the kidneys, prostaglandins maintain afferent arteriolar dilatation regulating renal blood flow and glomerular filtration rate. They also have a role in control of renin release and maintenance of water balance. NSAID inhibition of prostaglandin synthesis will result in reduction of renal blood flow and disrupt normal renal function and homeostatic mechanisms. Constriction of renal arterioles may result in renal papillary necrosis. These effects may be more evident in animals that are dehydrated or volume-depleted.

Kinetics and metabolism

Ibuprofen is completely absorbed in dogs. Absorption also occurs more rapidly than in humans, with peak plasma levels being achieved between 30 minutes and 3 hours. It is largely bound to serum proteins once absorbed (96%). The elimination half-life is between 2.5 and 5.4 hours. Inactive metabolites produced in the liver are excreted in the urine.

Clinical effects

The initial clinical effects usually occur within 2 hours. These include vomiting (often persistent), haematemesis, diarrhoea, melena, abdominal tenderness and anorexia. Mucous membranes may be pale or congested. Weakness, ataxia, incoordination, lethargy, depression and drowsiness are often noted. On rare occasions dyspnoea, hyperventilation, and tachycardia have been reported. Vocalisation, agitation, hyperactivity, hyperaesthesia, tremors, twitching or convulsions are occasionally observed. Coma has been reported in one VPISLn case (92/92984).

From 12 hours post-dose onwards, evidence of gastrointestinal irritation and renal impairment occurs. There may be protracted vomiting, pyrexia, anaemia, anorexia, polyuria, polydipsia, dehydration and collapse.

Renal impairment or failure should be anticipated if a dose of 250 mg/kg body weight has been exceeded. Initially this is characterised by oliguria, azotemia, and elevated creatinine and BUN. Such effects have been noted in some VPISLn cases (94/107678, 94/142289 and 94/149382). There may be hyperkalaemia and acidosis. Renal failure may be delayed for up to 5 days. Hypotensive or dehydrated animals are more at risk from renal effects, as are those with pre-existing renal impairment.

Gastric erosion, ulceration and, theoretically, perforation may occur, with doses as small as 8 mg/kg body weight This may occur in the absence of any major clinical effects. Dark, tarry stools may be observed in some animals with gastric ulceration (VPISLn cases 95/31770 and 95/29257).

Post-mortem findings

There may be evidence of gastrointestinal congestion and/or haemorrhage, gastric ulceration or perforation and renal tubule papillary necrosis.

Treatment

Treatment is advocated if a dose of 10 mg/kg body weight has been exceeded (5 mg/kg body weight in animals who are dehydrated, hypotensive or have pre-existing renal insufficiency).

If within 3 hours of ingestion, induce vomiting or perform gastric lavage, and then administer adsorbents.

Emetics:

(a)	Apomorphine	Dose:	0.05 mg/kg body weight i.v. or i.m.; 0.1 mg/kg body weight s.c.
(b)	Xylazine	Dose:	0.2 mg/kg body weight i.v.; 0.5–1 mg/kg body weight i.m. or s.c.
(c)	Ipecacuanha	Dose:	1–2 ml/kg body weight (maximum 20 ml) orally
(d)	Soda crystal.		

Adsorbents:

(a)	Activated charcoal	Dose:	2 g/kg body weight orally
(b)	BCK granules®	Dose:	6–18 g orally two or three times daily.

If there is severe or persistent vomiting then anti-emetics should be administered. If adsorbents have been administered this may reduce efficacy of orally administered anti-emetics. In such cases, parenteral administration is preferable. Either metoclopramide or acepromazine may be used; the latter has a longer duration of action.

(a)	Metoclopramide	Dose:	0.5–1 mg/kg body weight orally, s.c. or i.m. every 6–8 hours; 1–2 mg/kg body weight per day by slow i.v. infusion
(b)	Acepromazine	Dose:	0.03–0.1 mg/kg body weight i.v., i.m., or s.c. (use lower dose if giving i.v.); 1–3 mg/kg body weight orally.

Gastric effects

In *all* cases where treatment has been necessary, the animals should be administered ulcer-healing or ulcer-preventing drugs.

The H_2-receptor blocking drugs cimetidine, ranitidine and famotidine reduce gastric acid and pepsin secretions, reducing the risk of ulcer formation and allowing ulcers to heal. Omeprazole inhibits the proton pump responsible for gastric acid production by the parietal cells. It is more potent and has a longer duration of action (>24 hours) than the three aforementioned H_2-receptor blockers and its use should be reserved for animals who are not responding to other therapies.

Sucralfate is an ulcer-coating agent that binds to proteins at an ulcer site, protecting it from further gastric acid and pepsin attack.

Misoprostol is a synthetic prostaglandin analogue that in effect replaces the prostaglandins whose production is inhibited by ibuprofen. Administration shortly after ibuprofen ingestion will therefore ensure continued control of gastric acid secretion and increased mucous production, thereby preventing ulcer formation. Its use is contraindicated in animals who have already developed ulcers following NSAID ingestion.

Suggested regimen

The following treatment protocol is recommended for a 14-day period.

Either

| Cimetidine | Dose: | 5–10 mg/kg body weight i.v., i.m. or orally every 6–8 hours. |

Notes

1. If adsorbents have been administered then parenteral routes should be employed in the initial stages.
2. If the i.v. route is to be used then administer by slow i.v. injection over 30 minutes, to reduce risk of hypotension and arrhythmias.
3. If metoclopramide has been used or sucralfate is to be used then a period of 2 hours should elapse before cimetidine is administered.
4. Adverse effect – cimetidine blocks liver microsomal enzymes and therefore hepatic drug metabolism.

Or

| Ranitidine | Dose: | 0.5–4 mg/kg body weight i.v., s.c. or orally every 12 hours. |

Notes

1. If adsorbents have been administered then parenteral routes should be employed in the initial stages.
2. If metoclopramide has been used or sucralfate is to be used then a period of 2 hours should elapse before ranitidine is administered.

Or

| Famotidine | Dose: | 500 μg/kg body weight orally every 12 hours. |

Notes

1. Where adsorbents have been administered, a period of 2 hours should elapse before famotidine is administered, to minimise charcoal binding to drug.
2. If sucralfate is to be used then a period of 2 hours should elapse before famotidine is administered.

Where ingestion was recent and >10 mg/kg body weight of ibuprofen may have been ingested, also give:

| Misoprostol | Dose: | 1–5 μg/kg body weight orally every 6–8 hours for 24 hours. |

Notes

1. Where adsorbents have been administered, a period of 2 hours should elapse before misoprostol is administered, to minimise charcoal binding to drug.
2. If ulceration is already suspected or confirmed, misoprostol should not be given and sucralfate given instead.

3. Adverse effects – misoprostol may cause vomiting, diarrhoea and abdominal tenderness, and abortions in pregnant animals.

Where >10 mg/kg body weight ibuprofen may have been ingested and ulceration is either suspected or confirmed, give:

Sucralfate	Dose:	in dogs <20 kg body weight 500 mg/dog orally every 6–8 hours; in dogs >20 kg body weight 1 g/dog orally every 6–8 hours.

Notes

1. Where adsorbents have been administered, a period of 2 hours should elapse before sucralfate is administered, to minimise charcoal binding to drug.
2. If cimetidine, ranitidine or famotidine are to be used then sucralfate should be given 2 hours beforehand, as it requires an acid environment for maximum efficacy.
3. Ideally, sucralfate should be administered on an empty stomach, at least 1 hour prior to food.

If the animal does not respond to the above therapies then administration of omeprazole may be considered. The recommended dose is 0.5–1.5 mg/kg body weight orally every 24 hours.

Other care

Management is otherwise largely symptomatic and supportive. Ensure adequate hydration and good urine output. In some cases, dopamine may be necessary to increase renal perfusion and to minimise renal insufficiency (dose: 1–3 μg/kg body weight per minute as constant i.v. infusion).

If possible, blood gases and electrolytes should be checked and corrected, especially if there is evidence of renal dysfunction and/or oliguria. Bicarbonate should be given to correct acidosis. *Caution* – dopamine precipitates in bicarbonate solutions, so these fluids should not be administered together. If the animal is hyperkalaemic then this should be corrected using dextrose (dose: 20% solution given 1 ml/kg body weight i.v.), together with insulin if available (dose: 0.5 units/kg body weight).

Diazepam may be given if there is any convulsant activity (dose: 0.5 mg/kg body weight i.v., repeated every 10 minutes up to three times if needed).

Bland diets are recommended.

Enhanced elimination

Ibuprofen is protein-bound and extensively metabolised and therefore alkaline diuresis or urine alkalinisation, dialysis or haemoperfusion are unlikely to enhance elimination.

Investigative

Blood ibuprofen levels are not helpful in management except as confirmation of ingestion. Interpretation of levels is difficult and case management is better based on clinical condition of the animal. In any event, such analysis is not routinely offered by many laboratories.

In severe cases, radiography or gastroscopy may be employed to assess gastric mucosal damage.

Increases in prothrombin time or INR are rarely noted in ibuprofen overdoses.

In some VPISLn cases (94/107678, 94/142289 and 94/149382), elevated liver enzymes, BUN and creatinine have been recorded.

References and further reading

VPIS (London) past cases up to 97/12582.

Adams SS *et al.* (1969). Absorption, distribution and toxicity of ibuprofen. *Toxicology and Applied Pharmacology* **15**, 310–330.

Campbell A (1992). Ibuprofen in dogs – an example of species toxicity variation. Poster presentation for European Association of Poisons Centres and Clinical Toxicologists XV Congress, Istanbul, 24–27 May, 1992.

Earl JA (1987). Flurbiprofen warning. *Veterinary Record* **120**, 349.

Elliott GA (1988). The propionic acids. Gastrointestinal toxicity in various species. *Toxicologic Pathology* **16(2)**, 245–250.

England CGW (1987). Suspected flurbiprofen toxicity and its treatment in a dog. *Veterinary Record* **120**, 599–600.

Godshalk CP *et al.* (1992). Gastric perforation associated with administration of ibuprofen in a dog. *Journal of the American Veterinary Medical Association* **201(11)**, 1734–1736.

Jackson TW *et al.* (1991). Correlation of serum ibuprofen concentration with clinical signs of toxicity in three canine exposures. *Veterinary and Human Toxicology* **33(5)**, 486–488.

Jones RD *et al.* (1992). Non-steroidal anti-inflammatory drug toxicosis in dogs and cats: 240 cases. *Journal of the American Veterinary Medical Association* **201(3)**, 475–478.

Kore AM (1990). Toxicology of non-steroidal anti-inflammatory drugs. *Veterinary Clinics of North America: Small Animal Practice* **20**, 419–429.

Kore AM (1997). Over-the-counter analgesic drug toxicoses in small animals. *Veterinary Medicine* **92(2)**, 158–165.

Lascelles D and Balmer T (1997). Are all NSAIDs the same? *Veterinary Times* **24(4)**, 34–37.

Marlow CA (1987). Flurbiprofen warning. *Veterinary Record* **120**, 287.

Nash AS (1987). Flurbiprofen warning. *Veterinary Record* **120**, 399.

Poortinga EW and Hungerford LL (1998). A case–control study of acute ibuprofen toxicity in dogs. *Preventative Veterinary Medicine* **35(2)**, 115–124.

Sherkl R *et al.* (1987). Pharmacokinetics of ibuprofen in the dog. *Journal of Veterinary Pharmacology and Therapeutics* **10**, 261–265.

Smith KJ and Taylor DH (1993). Another case of gastric perforation associated with ibuprofen administration in a dog. *Journal of the American Veterinary Medical Association* **202(5)**, 706.

Spyridakis LK *et al.* (1986). Ibuprofen toxicosis in a dog. *Journal of the American Veterinary Medical Association* **188(9)**, 918–919.

Thursby-Pelham C (1996). Peculiar drug poisonings in pets. *In Practice* **18(10)**, 478–487.

Villar D, Buck WB and Gonzalez JM (1998). Ibuprofen, aspirin and acetaminophen toxicosis and treatment in dogs and cats. *Veterinary and Human Toxicology* **40(3)**, 156–161.

Vollmar AM (1993). Clinico-toxicologic aspects of non-steroidal anti-inflammatory agents in the dog and cat. *Tierarztliche Praxis* **21(2)**, 149–152 (in German).

Woolliscroft G and McArthur S (1987). Flurbiprofen toxicity in a dog. *Veterinary Record* **121**, 115–116.

Yeatts J (1988). Flurbiprofen toxicity. *Veterinary Record* **122**, 215.

Indomethacin

Type of product

Indomethacin is a non-steroidal, anti-inflammatory drug (NSAID) with antipyretic and analgesic activity.

Presentation

Indomethacin is available in the UK as a 'prescription only' medicine for human use. It is indicated for use in the management of pain and severe inflammation in rheumatic diseases, gout, musculoskeletal disorders, dysmenorrhoea and closure of the ductus arteriosus. It is sold under various brand names in tablet, capsule, liquid suspensions, and suppository preparations.

The dose of indomethacin in tablet and capsule preparations is variable but commonly 25 mg, 50 mg, and 75 mg. Some of these are modified- or sustained-release preparations.

Suppository preparations contain 100 mg of indomethacin and the liquid suspensions are commonly of 25 mg/5 ml strengths.

Occurrence of poisoning incidences

Since the launch of the VPIS in 1992, there have been a few enquiries about indomethacin ingestion by dogs each year. Half of these have developed clinical effects, but to date there have been no fatal outcomes to any of these cases.

Recommended dosage

In the UK, the drug is supplied for use in humans only. There are *no* indications for use of this drug in veterinary medicine. In dogs, its use is potentially dangerous.

Toxicity

Dogs are generally sensitive to NSAIDs, and although indomethacin is acetic acid derived, rather than propionic acid derived, clinical manifestations of adverse effects may be anticipated after ingestion of the drug. As with other NSAIDs, indomethacin causes severe gastrointestinal irritation and may also impair renal function at high doses.

According to the literature:

● There is no LD_{50} reported for dogs.

- Experimental dosings of 2 mg/kg body weight for 30 days caused ulcers in 60% of dogs and perforation in 20%. Increased doses of 3, 4 and 5 mg/kg over a similar period caused ulceration in all dogs and increasing perforation (50%, 70% and 90%, respectively). All the dogs given 2 mg/kg body weight survived. With the larger doses, survival time decreased with increasing dose.

In the experience of the VPISLn:

- Acute doses of 2.7 mg/kg body weight and 5 mg/kg caused no clinical effects in two cases (VPISLn cases 94/116351 and 94/60068).
- A single acute dose of 71 mg/kg body weight caused gastrointestinal irritation with no bleeding (VPISLn case 92/85934).
- 1.9 mg/kg body weight twice daily for 5 days caused gastrointestinal bleeding and renal dysfunction (VPISLn case 95/156181).

Case report

A dose of 25 mg (0.74 mg/kg body weight) of indomethacin in the evening and another 25 mg the following morning resulted in hospitalisation 24 hours later, with a 12-hour history of haematemesis, melena, anorexia and depression. The dog, a 34 kg bitch, also regularly received aspirin for osteoarthritis. On examination she was dehydrated, with abdominal pain. Barium contrast radiography revealed severe gastritis. She was discharged after 3 days of supportive care, but 24 hours later was readmitted with haematemesis and melena. Repeat barium contrast radiography again revealed severe gastritis. She vomited intermittently for 4 more days and diarrhoea and melena continued for almost 4 weeks. She lost 7 kg in weight but eventually began to improve and was discharged 35 days after the first attendance. She returned to hospital 1 month after this with anorexia and occasional vomiting and diarrhoea. She now weighed 25 kg. Laboratory analyses and barium contrast radiograph were normal. A surgical exploration of the abdomen was undertaken. Only the stomach was abnormal, with hyperaemia of the distal fundus and pyloric antrum. Partly digested blood (about 10 ml) was also present. A partial gastrectomy was performed, removing all the visible erosions. She made a good recovery and was discharged. Then, 131 days after the first admission (56 days after surgery) she again returned to hospital with haematemesis, diarrhoea, melena and complete anorexia. She weighed 28 kg. A barium contrast radiograph revealed adhesions between the duodenum and right dorsal abdominal wall. Surgical exploration revealed splenomegaly, and gastric and duodenal hyperaemia. She recovered well and was finally discharged 150 days after the first admission. She continued to have periods of vomiting, diarrhoea, anorexia, haematemesis and melena but recovered all her lost weight. Other causes of chronic haemorrhagic gastritis were ruled out. The fact that she regularly received aspirin may have made her more susceptible to the ulcerogenic potential of indomethacin (Ewing, 1972).

Mechanism of toxicity

Like other NSAIDs, indomethacin inhibits the cyclo-oxygenase step of prostaglandin synthesis. Such inhibition and subsequent reduction in levels of PGI_2 and PGE_2 can account for the major effects seen in poisoning cases.

In the gastrointestinal tract prostaglandins have a cytoprotective function, as they control production of gastric acid, stimulate secretion of mucous and bicarbonate by the gastric epithelium and maintain mucosal blood flow by causing vasodilatation. Deficiency will result in increased gastric acid secretion and reduction in mucous production and mucosal blood flow and therefore potentially lead to cell damage.

In the kidneys, prostaglandins maintain afferent arteriolar dilatation, regulating renal blood flow and glomerular filtration rate. They also have a role in control of renin release and maintenance of water balance. NSAID inhibition of prostaglandin synthesis will result in reduction of renal blood flow and disrupt normal renal function and homeostatic mechanisms. Constriction of renal arterioles may result in renal papillary necrosis. These effects may be more evident in animals that are dehydrated or volume depleted.

Kinetics and metabolism

Indomethacin appears to be rapidly absorbed in dogs. It is metabolised to form various metabolites in the liver that are excreted in the urine.

Clinical effects

The clinical effects usually occur within 2 hours following acute exposures. These include vomiting (often persistent), diarrhoea, abdominal tenderness and anorexia. Mucous membranes may be pale or congested. Weakness, lethargy, depression and drowsiness are possible effects.

From 12 hours post-dose onwards, evidence of gastrointestinal irritation and renal impairment may occur, particularly after large acute ingestions or repeated low doses. There may be protracted vomiting, pyrexia, anorexia, polyuria, polydipsia, dehydration, renal dysfunction and collapse. Hypotensive or dehydrated animals are more at risk from renal effects, as are those with pre-existing renal impairment.

Gastric erosion, ulceration and, theoretically, perforation with intestinal irritation will occur, with large acute dosings, or repeated doses above 2 mg/kg body weight per day. This may occur in the absence of any major clinical effects. Dark, tarry stools may be observed in some animals with gastric ulceration.

Post-mortem findings

There may be evidence of gastrointestinal congestion and/or haemorrhage, gastric ulceration or perforation and renal tubule papillary necrosis.

Treatment

Treatment is advocated if a single acute dose of 10 mg/kg body weight has been exceeded (5 mg/kg body weight in animals who are dehydrated, hypotensive or have pre-existing renal insufficiency).

If within 3 hours of ingestion, induce vomiting or perform gastric lavage, and then administer adsorbents.

Emetics:

(a) Apomorphine	Dose:	0.05 mg/kg body weight i.v. or i.m.; 0.1 mg/kg body weight s.c.	
(b) Xylazine	Dose:	0.2 mg/kg body weight i.v.; 0.5–1 mg/kg body weight i.m. or s.c.	
(c) Ipecacuanha	Dose:	1–2 ml/kg body weight (maximum 20 ml) orally	
(d) Soda crystal.			

Adsorbents:

(a) Activated charcoal	Dose:	2 g/kg body weight orally
(b) BCK granules®	Dose:	6–18 g orally two or three times daily.

If there is severe or persistent vomiting then anti-emetics should be administered. If adsorbents have been administered this may reduce efficacy of orally administered anti-emetics. In such cases, parenteral administration is preferable. Either metoclopramide or acepromazine may be used; the latter has a longer duration of action.

(a) Metoclopramide	Dose:	0.5–1 mg/kg body weight orally, s.c. or i.m. every 6–8 hours; 1–2 mg/kg body weight per day by slow i.v. infusion
(b) Acepromazine	Dose:	0.03–0.1 mg/kg body weight i.v., i.m., or s.c. (use lower dose if giving i.v.); 1–3 mg/kg body weight orally.

Gastric effects

In *all* cases where treatment has been necessary, the animals should be administered ulcer-healing or ulcer-preventing drugs.

The H$_2$-receptor blocking drugs cimetidine, ranitidine and famotidine reduce gastric acid and pepsin secretions, reducing risk of ulcer formation and allowing ulcers to heal. Omeprazole inhibits the proton pump responsible for gastric acid production by the parietal cells. It is more potent and has a longer duration of action (> 24 hours) than the three aforementioned H_2-receptor blockers and its use should be reserved for animals who are not responding to other therapies.

Sucralfate is an ulcer-coating agent that binds to proteins at an ulcer site, protecting it from further gastric acid and pepsin attack.

Misoprostol is a synthetic prostaglandin analogue that in effect replaces the prostaglandins whose production is inhibited by NSAIDs. Administration shortly after NSAID ingestion will therefore ensure continued control of gastric acid secretion and increased mucous production, thereby preventing ulcer formation. Its use is contraindicated in animals who have already developed ulcers following NSAID ingestion.

Suggested regimen

The following treatment protocol is recommended for a 14-day period.

Either

Cimetidine   Dose: 5–10 mg/kg body weight i.v., i.m. or orally every 6–8 hours.

Notes

1. If adsorbents have been administered then parenteral routes should be employed in the initial stages.
2. If the i.v. route is to be used then administer by slow i.v. injection over 30 minutes to reduce risk of hypotension and arrhythmias.
3. If metoclopramide has been used or sucralfate is to be used then a period of 2 hours should elapse before cimetidine is administered.
4. Adverse effect – cimetidine blocks liver microsomal enzymes and therefore hepatic drug metabolism.

Or

Ranitidine   Dose: 0.5–4 mg/kg body weight i.v., s.c. or orally every 12 hours.

Notes

1. If adsorbents have been administered then parenteral routes should be employed in the initial stages.
2. If metoclopramide has been used or sucralfate is to be used then a period of two hours should elapse before ranitidine is administered.

Or

Famotidine   Dose: 500 μg/kg body weight orally every 12 hours.

Notes

1. Where adsorbents have been administered, a period of 2 hours should elapse before famotidine is administered, to minimise binding to drug.

2. If sucralfate is to be used then a period of 2 hours should elapse before famotidine is administered.

Where ingestion was recent, also give:

Misoprostol   Dose: 1–5 µg/kg body weight orally every 6–8 hours for 24 hours.

Notes

1. Where adsorbents have been administered, a period of 2 hours should elapse before misoprostol is administered, to minimise binding to drug.
2. If ulceration is already suspected or confirmed, misoprostol should not be given and sucralfate given instead.
3. Adverse effects – misoprostol may cause vomiting, diarrhoea and abdominal tenderness, and abortions in pregnant animals.

Where ulceration is either suspected or confirmed, give:

Sucralfate   Dose: in dogs <20 kg body weight 500 mg/dog orally every 6–8 hours; in dogs >20 kg body weight 1 g/dog orally every 6–8 hours.

Notes

1. Where adsorbents have been administered, a period of 2 hours should elapse before sucralfate is administered, to minimise binding to drug.
2. If cimetidine, ranitidine or famotidine are to be used then sucralfate should be given 2 hours beforehand, as it requires an acid environment for maximum efficacy.
3. Ideally, sucralfate should be administered on an empty stomach, at least 1 hour prior to food.

If the animal does not respond to the above therapies then administration of omeprazole may be considered. The recommended dose is 0.5–1.5 mg/kg body weight orally every 24 hours.

Other care

Management is otherwise largely symptomatic and supportive. Ensure adequate hydration and good urine output. In some cases, dopamine may be necessary to increase renal perfusion and to minimise renal insufficiency (dose: 1–3 µg/kg body weight per minute as constant i.v. infusion).

If possible, blood gases and electrolytes should be checked and corrected, especially if there is evidence of renal dysfunction and/or oliguria. Bicarbonate should be given to correct acidosis. *Caution* – dopamine precipitates in bicarbonate solutions, so these fluids should not be administered together. If the animal is hyperkalaemic then this should be corrected using dextrose (dose: 20% solution given 1 ml/kg body weight i.v.), together with insulin if available (dose: 0.5 units/kg body weight).

Diazepam may be given if there is any convulsant activity. Dose: 0.5 mg/kg body weight i.v. repeated every 10 minutes up to three times if needed.

Bland diets are recommended.

Enhanced elimination

Alkaline diuresis or urine alkalinisation, dialysis or haemoperfusion are unlikely to enhance elimination.

Investigative

Blood indomethacin levels are not helpful in management, except as confirmation of ingestion. Interpretation of levels is difficult and case management is better based on the clinical condition of the animal. In any event, such analysis is not routinely offered by many laboratories.

In severe cases, radiography or gastroscopy may be employed to assess gastric mucosal damage.

References and further reading

VPIS (London) past cases up to 96/160278.

Ewing GO (1972). Indomethacin-associated gastrointestinal hemorrhage in a dog. *Journal of the American Veterinary Medical Association* **161(12)**, 1665–1668.

Horton R and Zisper R (1978). Prostaglandins: renin release and renal function. *Contributions to Nephrology* **14**, 87–96.

Jones RD et al. (1992). Non-steroidal anti-inflammatory drug toxicosis in dogs and cats: 240 cases. *Journal of the American Veterinary Medical Association* **201(3)**, 475–478.

Kore AM (1990). Toxicology of non-steroidal anti-inflammatory drugs. *Veterinary Clinics of North America: Small Animal Practice* **20**, 419–429.

Kore AM (1997). Over-the-counter analgesic drug toxicoses in small animals. *Veterinary Medicine* **92(2)**, 158–165.

Lascelles D and Balmer T (1997). Are all NSAIDs the same? *Veterinary Times* **24(4)**, 34–37.

Nicoloff DM (1968). Indomethacin – Effect on gastric secretion, parietal cell population and ulcer provocation in the dog. *Archives of Surgery* **97**, 809–815.

Vollar AM (1993). Clinico-toxicologic aspects of non-steroidal anti-inflammatory agents in the dog and cat. *Tierarztliche Praxis* **21(2)**, 149–152 (in German).

Iron and iron salts

Type of product

Iron salts are used in man as dietary supplements for the treatment of iron deficiency. Some multivitamin and mineral supplement preparations also contain small quantities of iron, usually present as the sulphate.

Iron salts are also present in some lawn moss killers.

Presentation
Pharmaceutical

In dietary supplements and multivitamin preparations the sulphate, fumarate and gluconate are the commonly encountered salts. Some of the preparations are sustained- or modified-release varieties.

Ferrous sulphate

Usually available in tablet, capsule or spansule preparations of strengths 150 mg (47 mg elemental iron), 160 mg (50 mg elemental iron), 200 mg (65 mg elemental iron) and 325 mg (105 mg elemental iron).

An oral solution of ferrous sulphate for paediatric use is available, which contains 60 mg/5 ml (12 mg elemental iron/5 ml).

Ferrous fumarate

Usually available in tablet, capsule or spansule preparations of strengths 200 mg (65 mg elemental iron), 305 mg (100 mg elemental iron), 322 mg (100 mg elemental iron) and 330 mg (110 mg elemental iron).

An oral solution of ferrous fumarate is available, which contains 140 mg/5 ml (45 mg elemental iron/5 ml).

Ferrous gluconate

Usually available in tablet, capsule or spansule preparations of strengths 250 mg (30 mg elemental iron) and 300 mg (35 mg elemental iron).

An oral solution of ferrous fumarate is available, which contains 140 mg/5 ml (45 mg elemental iron/5 ml).

Agricultural

Some lawn sands or moss killers contain up to 30% w/w or w/v ferrous sulphate. For a 30% strength preparation 1 kg or 1 litre of product would contain the equivalent of 97.5 g of elemental iron.

Occurrence of poisoning incidences

Since the launch of the VPIS, up to 20 enquiries per annum have involved canine ingestion of iron salts as a pharmaceutical and up to eight as a component of a lawn sand or moss killer. A small percentage of these have developed clinical effects. One fatal case has been recorded. This was due to ingestion of a lawn sand preparation.

Recommended dosage

For treatment and prevention of iron-deficiency anaemia – ferrous sulphate: 100–300 mg orally once daily or iron dextran: 25 mg/kg body weight i.m. weekly as required.

Toxicity

According to the literature:

- The oral LD_{50} in dogs for ferrous sulphate is 600 mg/kg body weight.
- The intravenous LD_{50} of ferrous sulphate in dogs is 79 mg/kg body weight.
- Ingested doses greater than 20 mg/kg body weight elemental iron are considered moderately toxic.
- Ingested doses greater than 200 mg/kg body weight elemental iron are potentially lethal.

In the experience of the VPISLn:

- There have been no fatal cases resulting from ingestion of pharmaceutical preparations.
- Doses equivalent to 18 mg/kg body weight of elemental iron have caused mild gastrointestinal effects.
- 36 mg/kg body weight equivalent of elemental iron resulted in no clinical effects.
- 171 mg/kg body weight equivalent of elemental iron resulted in severe abdominal tenderness and dark-coloured faeces at 24 hours post-ingestion in a German Shepherd dog. The animal was treated with intravenous fluids and desferrioxamine and made a full recovery (VPISLn case 94/135340).
- An estimated dose of 866 mg/kg body weight of elemental iron (ingested as fumarate) resulted in severe and protracted vomiting in a West Highland terrier. No treatment was given but the animal developed no other clinical effects (VPISLn case 92/74040).
- A German Shepherd cross-bred dog ate an unknown quantity of a lawn sand containing ferrous sulphate. The animal developed lethargy, pale mucous membranes, severe vomiting, diarrhoea, melena and collapsed. Despite aggressive management with intravenous fluid therapy, multivitamins and desferrioxamine, the animal died. Post-

mortem analysis confirmed death due to iron poisoning (VPISLn case 96/145380).

Mechanism of toxicity

Under normal conditions, the amount of iron absorbed from the diet is determined by the body's iron requirement, with absorption taking place via an active process in the mucosal cells of the duodenum and jejunum. Absorbed iron is bound to transferrin and transported to the reticulo-endothelial system, bone marrow and hepatocytes, where it is stored and utilised. There is no specific mechanism for the excretion of iron. An excessive intake of iron overwhelms the selective transport mechanism and excess circulates as free iron.

Iron salts are corrosive and cause direct damage to cells. Gastrointestinal perforation and peritonitis are therefore possible. Mitochondrial damage causes hepatic necrosis, and increased capillary permeability and post-arteriolar dilatation can lead to cardiovascular collapse. Also, free-radical formation is enhanced with increased iron availability and may result in additional cell damage.

Kinetics and metabolism

Iron salts are rapidly absorbed from the gastrointestinal tract.

Clinical effects

Following ingestion, the initial signs usually occur within 6 hours and include buccal irritation, vomiting, haematemesis, haemorrhagic diarrhoea, drowsiness, weakness, and depression. There may then be apparent recovery over 6–24 hours. This may be followed by dehydration, shock, renal failure (secondary to shock), liver damage and coma. Haemoglobinaemia and coagulopathy may occur.

Laboratory diagnosis

- Elevated serum iron levels.
- Metabolic acidosis.
- Elevated LFTs and bilirubin.

The normal serum iron concentration in dogs is 17–22 μmol/L (94–122 μg/dl).

There are no definite data on toxic serum iron levels in dogs, although levels greater than 62 μmol/L (350 μg/dl) are considered dangerous.

Post-mortem findings

Common findings include mucosal necrosis and ulceration, enteritis, liver necrosis and congestion of splanchnic vessels, liver and kidney.

Treatment

Treatment is advised if more than the equivalent of 30 mg/kg body weight of elemental iron has been consumed.

Undissolved iron tablets are radio-opaque and X-ray may therefore be used to confirm ingestion. However, absence of radio-opaque material does not exclude ingestion.

If within 3 hours of ingestion, induce vomiting or perform gastric lavage.

Emetics:

(a) Apomorphine	Dose:	0.05 mg/kg body weight i.v. or i.m.; 0.1 mg/kg body weight s.c.
(b) Xylazine	Dose:	0.2 mg/kg body weight i.v.; 0.5–1 mg/kg body weight i.m. or s.c.
(c) Ipecacuanha	Dose:	1–2 ml/kg body weight (maximum 20 ml) orally
(d) Soda crystal.		

Iron is not adsorbed to activated charcoal and therefore the use of adsorbents is not recommended.

Elimination techniques

A chelating agent, desferrioxamine, is available for the management of iron poisoning. The drug chelates free iron, removing it from cellular binding sites, and the resultant complex is excreted in the urine, turning it a pink-brown colour.

In dogs, it should be given if there are definite signs of poisoning or where a large amount is thought to have been ingested. It should also be used if the serum iron concentration is greater than 60 μmol/L (335 μg/dl). In practice it may be difficult to obtain a serum iron level in time to determine this need and in many cases desferrioxamine is given anyway.

Desferrioxamine dose: 40 mg/kg body weight i.v. *slowly* over 4 hours. Note: Rapid administration of desferrioxamine may cause hypotension or cardiac arrhythmias.

- If the dog remains asymptomatic and the urine is the normal colour, no further doses are required.
- If the dog is symptomatic and/or the urine is a pink-brown colour then further doses should be given every 4–6 hours.

Management is otherwise supportive, with particular care required to ensure adequate hydration.

Reference

VPIS (London) past cases up to 97/86932.

Ivermectin

Type of product

Ivermectin is an antiparasitic agent and is one of the avermectins. These are natural or semi-natural macrocyclic lactone disaccharides that are fermentation products of *Streptomyces avermitilis* and *Streptomyces cyamogriseus*. Ivermectin is a mixture of about 80% 22,23-dihydroavermectin B_{1a} and 20% 22,23-dihydroavermectin B_{1b}. It is active against mature and immature nematodes and arthropods.

It has veterinary use for the control of migrating heartworm (*Dirofilaria immitis*) larvae in dogs. This nematode worm is not endemic in the UK, but may be present in some quarantine dogs. It is also used for management of intractable dermal parasiticoses.

Ivermectin is used for control of gastrointestinal roundworms and lungworms in horses, ruminants and pigs; type II ostertagiasis in ruminants; horse bots; some lice and mites on cattle and pigs; warble fly larvae in cattle; nasal bots in sheep; and mites on cats.

Presentations

Several preparations are available but none specifically for dogs, since ivermectin is not licensed in the UK for use against heartworm in dogs. In, non-canine farm animals, ivermectin may be given orally, subcutaneously or as a pour-on application. Oral preparations may be pastes or liquids and can contain up to 20 mg/dose or up to 1 mg/ml, respectively. Preparations for injection are available at 10 mg/ml strength and pour-on solutions at 5 mg/ml. Dogs usually ingest one of the oral preparations.

Some modified-release ruminal preparations for cattle are available, designed to release 1.72 g over 135 days.

Occurrence of poisoning incidences

Since 1992, the VPIS London centre has received between five and 10 enquiries per annum regarding ivermectin exposures in dogs. Many of the cases involve collie breeds, who have inadvertently drunk preparations intended for use in other animals. Two fatal cases have been reported, both following injection (VPISLn cases 95/65270 and 96/39127).

Recommended dosage

In the UK, ivermectin is not licensed for use against heartworm in dogs. However 'off label' use for management of dermal parasite infections is common.

For heartworm prophylaxis, the recommended dosage in the USA is 6 μg/kg body weight orally every month.

In some UK formularies, a dose of 0.2 mg/kg body weight either s.c. or i.m. is quoted for dogs and cats. In some dogs, particularly collie breeds, such a dosing is likely to cause toxicity.

In general, doses less than 50 μg/kg body weight will be tolerated by most animals, although caution is recommended in neonatal animals and collie related breeds.

Toxicity

According to the literature:

- Doses less than 50 μg/kg body weight should not affect even sensitive breeds or species.
- 50–100 μg/kg body weight may cause adverse reactions in collie breeds.
- 200 μg/kg body weight causes convulsant-like activity, depression, muscle weakness, blindness, coma and death. Cases with ataxia often progress to paralysis and decreased consciousness.
- 200 μg/kg body weight ingested by a Collie caused salivation, ataxia and disorientation within 3 hours. Coma and respiratory failure followed. The dog was treated with i.v. fluids and anticholinergics. EKG showed no CNS involvement and the animal recovered over 14 days.
- Beagles receiving doses of 2.5 mg/kg body weight developed dilated pupils. A dose of 5–20 mg/kg body weight caused tremors and ataxia and 40 mg/kg body weight proved fatal.
- Oral LD_{50} in beagles is quoted as 80 mg/kg body weight.
- Beagles given 2 mg/kg acutely or 0.5 mg/kg daily for 14 weeks showed no toxic effects.
- A Doberman that had ingested 2.9 mg/kg body weight was found 24 hours later with recumbency, twitching, dilated pupils and dehydration. The animal was apparently blind. With supportive care the animal recovered over 8 days.
- An Old English Sheepdog-type dog ingesting 150 μg/kg body weight developed hind-limb ataxia, hypersalivation, hyperventilation, constricting pupils, extreme drowsiness, and loss of menace response.
- Pregnant bitches of unspecified breed were given 500 μg/kg body weight eight times between 5 and 40 days of gestation. No ivermectin-related effects were seen in either the bitches or the foetuses.

In the experience of the VPISLn:

- 140 µg/kg body weight ingested by a Rough Collie caused severe lethargy, ataxia, salivation, inappetence, polydipsia and sluggish pupil reflexes within 14 hours. The animal survived with supportive care (VPISLn case 91/90939)
- Another Rough Collie was inadvertently injected with 1 ml of a 10 mg/ml preparation intended for use in cattle. The animal became severely ataxic, with hyperventilation, and lethargy. Despite supportive care with rehydration, use of corticosteroids, antibiotics and millophylline, the animal died 12 days post-exposure (VPISLn case 95/65270).

Mechanism of toxicity

Avermectins interfere with parasite nerve transmission by increasing release of the inhibitory neurotransmitter gamma-aminobutyric acid (GABA) from pre-synaptic nerve terminals and enhancing binding to post-synaptic receptors. This leads to the opening of post-synaptic chloride channels, causing neuronal hyperpolarisation and depression of neuronal function. They may also act on chloride channels independent of GABA receptors. In invertebrates, where GABA receptors are found in the peripheral nervous system, this causes paralysis, cell dysfunction and death of the animal. In mammals, where GABA receptors are located in the CNS, the result of excess GABA release and post-synaptic binding would be diffuse cerebellar and cerebral cortex dysfunction. However, in mammals avermectins do not readily cross the blood–brain barrier and so toxicity is much reduced.

Collie breeds appear to have sensitivity to ivermectin because of an increased penetration of the CNS, which may be due to an increased permeability of their blood–brain barrier or to the existence of a transport mechanism for ivermectin across this barrier.

The reversible blindness seen in some canine ivermectin cases may be attributable to increased inhibitory activity, both pre- and post-synaptically, in the CNS. This blindness appears to occur even though the pupils respond to light stimulation.

Some authors suggest that a recessive autosomal gene may be responsible for the idiosyncratic reactions seen in collies.

Kinetics and metabolism

Ivermectin is well absorbed both orally (approximately 95%) and parenterally, and is concentrated in the fat and liver. In high dose, it crosses the blood–brain barrier. Peak plasma concentrations following oral exposures are achieved within 3–5 hours. Plasma concentrations do not correlate with neurological signs in either collie or non-collie breeds.

Ivermectin is metabolised in the liver into methyl alcohol and mono-saccharides and the majority of the metabolites are excreted in the faeces, with only 0.5–2% being excreted in the urine. It is also excreted in the milk of lactating animals.

Plasma half-life is approximately 2 days following oral administration.

Clinical effects

Some breeds are more susceptible to ivermectin toxicity, particularly Collies, Border Collies, and possibly Shelties, Australian Shepherd Dogs and related breeds. Even with susceptible breeds, there is wide variation in sensitivity between individual animals.

Onset of effects is usually within 4–6 hours of oral exposure, although in some cases effects are not observed until 10–14 hours post-exposure. Recovery may be protracted; in most cases, it occurs within 48 hours, although in some large exposures complete recovery has taken several weeks.

Cases where mild intoxication has occurred are characterised by constricted pupils, although some reported cases detail dilation of pupils, salivation, confusion, disorientation and lethargy. Pupil reflexes may be sluggish or absent. Some animals have been reported as polydipsic.

Severe intoxications are characterised by ataxia, vomiting, pin-point pupils, blindness, tremors, depression, convulsions, hyperaesthesia, tremors, hyperreflexia, hypothermia or hyperthermia, drowsiness, stupor, coma and paralysis. Rarely, bradycardia and respiratory depression are reported. Acidosis has occasionally been documented.

Note: rapid die-off of larvae in heartworm (*Dirofilaria immitus*)-infected dogs may cause vomiting, lethargy, tremor, tachycardia and shock.

Post-mortem findings

At post-mortem there are no diagnostic lesions observed in ivermectin-poisoned animals. In experimental cases, mild pulmonary congestion/oedema and focal CNS haemorrhage were found. However, these findings were not conclusively linked to ivermectin exposure.

Treatment

Treatment is recommended for doses >150 μg/kg body weight in susceptible breeds and for >2.5 mg/kg in non-susceptible breeds. These doses are given only as a guide, as some individual animals may exhibit toxicity at lower doses and merit treatment accordingly.

If within 3 hours of ingestion, induce vomiting or consider gastric lavage, and then administer adsorbents.

Emetics:

(a) Apomorphine	Dose:	0.05 mg/kg body weight i.v. or i.m.; 0.1 mg/kg body weight s.c.
(b) Xylazine	Dose:	0.2 mg/kg body weight i.v.; 0.5–1 mg/kg body weight i.m. or s.c.
(c) Ipecacuanha	Dose:	1–2 ml/kg body weight (maximum 20 ml) orally
(d) Soda crystal.		

Adsorbents:

(a) Activated charcoal	Dose:	2 g/kg body weight orally
(b) BCK granules®	Dose:	6–18 g orally two or three times daily.

Treatment is essentially symptomatic and supportive and most dogs recover with good nursing care. In particular, the monitoring of electrolytes and fluid balance, blood pressure, heart rate, body temperature, blood gases and respiratory function is advocated.

Animals with bradycardia may be given atropine or the muscarinic receptor antagonist glycopyrollate. The former is recommended for mild cases only as, unlike glycopyrollate, it will cross the blood–brain barrier, further compromising the neurological status of the animal.

Atropine dose: 30–50 μg/kg body weight s.c. or i.m.; 20 μg/kg body weight i.v. Glycopyrollate dose: 10 μg/kg body weight s.c.

Although there is no evidence of ivermectin causing cerebral oedema, some authors recommend use of dexamethasone in severe cases. Dose: 2–3 mg/kg body weight i.v. then 1 mg/kg body weight s.c. every 8 hours.

Cimetidine has been recommended to reduce gastric irritation. Dose: 5–10 mg/kg body weight i.v., i.m. or orally every 6–8 hours.

In severe cases, ventilation may be required for respiratory depression, and parenteral nutrition should be started as early as possible.

In severe cases where the animals have become unresponsive, the cholinesterase inhibitor physostigmine has been used. Physostigmine causes neuronal hypopolarisation by increasing sodium conductance at the post-synaptic nerve endings, thereby offsetting the effects of the chloride channel-mediated hyperpolarisation. The duration of action for physostigmine is short, with effects usually lasting less than 60 minutes. Use may be associated with development of convulsions.

Physostigmine dose: 0.6 mg/kg body weight by slow i.v. injection. Prior use of glycopyrollate to offset potential bradycardia should be considered.

Picrotoxin, a natural glucoside alkaloid that acts as an analeptic, has been suggested as possible antidote to ivermectin poisoning. It is a chloride channel blocker that functions as a GABA antagonist blocking post-synaptic hyperpolarisation. It has been used successfully in some serious cases but it is non-selective, has a narrow margin of safety, and its use is associated with development of convulsions. It therefore should not be routinely used for ivermectin poisoning cases.

Contra-indicated drugs

Benzodiazepine use is best avoided, as it also enhances CNS GABAergic activity, owing to ivermectin causing an increased affinity of benzodiazepines for the GABA receptor–chloride channel complex.

Investigations

Plasma levels may be useful in confirming ingestion and toxic exposures.

Heartworm-infested dogs

In infested dogs displaying adverse reactions, recommended management is essentially symptomatic and supportive with use of corticosteroids, fluid replacement and respiratory support as required.

References and further reading

VPIS (London) past cases up to 97/101602.

Campbell WC and Benz GW (1984). Ivermectin: a review of efficacy and safety. *Journal of Veterinary Pharmacology and Therapeutics* **7**, 1–16.

Fassler PE *et al.* (1991). Evaluation of the safety of ivermectin administered in a beef-based formulation to ivermectin-sensitive collies. *Journal of the American Veterinary Medical Association* **199(4)**, 457–460.

Hadrick MK *et al.* (1995). Ivermectin toxicosis in two Australian Shepherds. *Journal of the American Veterinary Medical Association* **206(8)**, 1147–1152.

Heit JE *et al.* (1989). Clinical management of ivermectin overdose in a Collie dog. *Companion Animal Practice – Toxicology*, **19(1)**, 3–7.

Hopkins KD *et al.* (1990). Ivermectin toxicosis in a dog. *Journal of the American Veterinary Medical Association* **197(1)**, 93–94.

Houston DM *et al.* (1987). Ivermectin toxicosis in a dog. *Journal of the American Veterinary Medical Association* **191**, 78.

Hsu WH *et al.* (1989). The safety of ivermectin. *Compendium of Continuing Education: Small Animal Practice* **11(5)**, 584–589.

Kieran P (1987). Toxicity associated with anthelmintics. In *Veterinary Clinical Toxicology, Proceedings No. 103* (Proceedings of a conference held at the University of Sydney, Australia, 24–28 August 1987), pp. 443–476.

Lovell RA (1990). Ivermectin and piperazine toxicoses in dogs and cats. *Veterinary Clinics of North America: Small Animal Practice* **20(2)**, 453–468.

Paradis M (1998). Ivermectin in small animal dermatology. Part 1. Pharmacology and Toxicology. *Compendium on Continuing Education for the Practising Veterinarian* **20(2)**, 193–200.

Paul AJ *et al.* (1987). Clinical observations in Collies given ivermectin orally. *American Journal of Veterinary Research* **48(4)**, 684–685.

Pulliam JD et al. (1985). Investigating ivermectin toxicity in Collies. Veterinary Medicine 80(6), 33–40.

Roder JD and Stair EL (1998). An overview of ivermectin toxicosis. Veterinary and Human Toxicology 40(6), 369–370.

Ryan WG and Jones PH (1989). Ivermectin use in Collie dogs. Veterinary Record 125(16), 425.

Seward RL (1983). Reactions in dogs given ivermectin. Journal of the American Veterinary Medical Association 183(5), 493.

Tranquilli WJ et al. (1987). Response to physostigmine administration in Collie dogs exhibiting ivermectin toxicosis. Journal of Veterinary Pharmacology and Therapeutics 10, 96–100.

Tranquilli WJ et al. (1989) Ivermectin plasma concentrations in Collies sensitive to ivermectin-induced toxicosis. American Journal of Veterinary Research 50(5), 769–770.

Wijnands-Kleukers AP et al. (1996). Ivermectin: Dangerous for dogs. Tijdschrift voor Diergeneeskunde 121(16), 446–448 (in Dutch).

Laburnum species

The plant

Common names are: Bean Tree, Golden Chain, Laburnum and Golden Rain. It is a member of the Leguminosae family.

Laburnum is a cultivated ornamental, sometimes found on waste ground as an escape from cultivation. It grows 7–9 m high. The leaves have long stalks with three terminal, oval leaflets, light green in colour and downy underneath. In summer, clusters of bright yellow flowers develop. These are borne on pendulous racemes 10–20 cm long. The seeds are contained in pods 3–5 cm long. Initially green with green seeds, they mature into pale brown, dry pods. Each pod holds between three and eight brown or black seeds.

Occurrence of poisoning incidences

Since 1992, the VPIS has received between five and 15 enquiries per year regarding laburnum ingestion. These cases have principally involved dogs, where pods, leaves and flowers have been consumed. No cases have had a fatal outcome, though some 70% have developed clinical effects.

Toxicity

All parts of the Laburnum are toxic. However, severe cases are relatively rare, probably as ingestion of large quantities usually results in emesis of rapid onset.

According to the literature:

- Toxicity has been reported in dogs following chewing of the twigs and bark.
- The fatal dose of seeds in a dog has been quoted as 6 g/kg (Clarke).
- Two cases of laburnum poisoning in dogs are reported. One 7-month-old English Setter bitch was treated for mild diarrhoea of 24 hours' duration. A kaolin and neomycin preparation was prescribed. The next day the bitch collapsed during normal exercise and died within 2 minutes. Post-mortem revealed an acute gastroenteritis, petechiation of the thymus and a large quantity of fine 2-inch long pods in the stomach; the significance of the stomach contents was not realised at the time. Two hours later, the second animal collapsed with marked muscle tremors, vomiting, and diarrhoea. Several treatments were initiated to cover all possibilities, although poisoning was suspected. The animal recovered. Three weeks later the dog collapsed again, although the other clinical effects were less marked. It was noted, that

the dogs used to chew the low hanging branches of a laburnum tree. After the tree was felled, no further episodes were reported (Leyland). In the experience of VPISLn:

- No fatal cases reported.
- A 2-month-old Dachshund puppy ingested laburnum flowers and developed vomiting. The dog was given adsorbents and made a quick recovery (VPISLn case 93/49336).
- A 25 kg Collie ate several laburnum pods. The animal developed severe muscle rigidity, especially in the hind legs, together with hyperaesthesia, facial spasms and dilated unreactive pupils. The animal was given diazepam and penicillin and made a gradual recovery over 3 days (VPISLn case 94/19569).
- A 26-month-old mongrel ate an unknown number of laburnum pods and leaves. The animal developed hyperaesthesia, ptosis, apparent blindness, diarrhoea and ataxia. The dog was given intravenous fluid support and atropine and made a full recovery (VPISLn case 97/78056).

Mechanism of toxicity

The main toxin in Laburnum species is cytisine, a quinolizidine alkaloid. All parts of the plant contain the alkaloid, so have a potential to cause toxicity. Cytisine has a nicotine-like action. Both nicotine and cytisine work on the same autonomic ganglia receptors. Cytisine is the more prominent respiratory stimulant and has a weaker curare-like action than nicotine.

Kinetics and metabolism

Cytisine is rapidly absorbed via the mucous membranes of the mouth. It is less well absorbed if the seeds are ingested intact. Peak plasma concentrations are seen at 2 hours post-oral dose in mice. It is excreted unchanged in the urine. Studies in mice found the half-life of cytisine to be approximately 200 minutes.

Clinical effects

The common effects are salivation, vomiting, and diarrhoea. These have a rapid onset. The centrally stimulated vomiting may persist for 1–2 days.

Listlessness, muscular spasms, and incoordination have also been reported in past VPIS cases. In severe cases, the central stimulation effects of cytisine cause delirium, excitation, tonic-clonic convulsions can occur. Death is usually due to respiratory paralysis.

Post-mortem findings

There are no characteristic findings on post-mortem. A post-mortem of a 7-month-old setter bitch showed acute gastroenteritis and petechiation of the thymus, and a large quantity of laburnum pods were found in the stomach.

Treatment

If the animal has not vomited and is presented to surgery within 2 hours of the ingestion then use of emesis and absorbents is recommended. Gastric lavage is probably unnecessary.

Emetics:

(a) Apomorphine	Dose:	0.05 mg/kg body weight i.v. or i.m.; 0.1 mg/kg body weight s.c.
(b) Xylazine	Dose:	0.2 mg/kg body weight i.v.; 0.5–1 mg/kg body weight i.m. or s.c.
(c) Ipecacuanha	Dose:	1–2 ml/kg body weight (maximum 20 ml) orally
(d) Soda crystal.		

Adsorbents:

(a) Activated charcoal	Dose:	2 g/kg body weight orally
(b) BCK granules®	Dose:	6–18 g orally two or three times daily.

Management thereafter is symptomatic and supportive, as there is no specific antidote. An minimum observation period of 6 hours post-ingestion is recommended. The animal should be kept well hydrated.

References

VPIS (London) past cases up to 97/78056.

Baker I (1993). Laburnum. *In Practice* **15(1)**, 20.

Clarke M (1993). Laburnum poisoning (letter). *In Practice* **15(2)**, 66.

Frohne D and Pfander HJ (1983). *A Colour Atlas of Poisonous Plants*. London: Wolfe Publishing, pp. 124–125.

Leyland A (1981). Laburnum (*Cytisus laburnum*) poisoning in two dogs. *Veterinary Record* **109**, 287.

Rose F (1991). *The Wild Flower Key*. London: Frederick Warne, pp. 180–181.

Loperamide

Type of product

Loperamide is a weak opioid with weak analgesic activity. It has licensed use in veterinary medicine as a treatment for non-specific chronic and acute diarrhoea. It also has human use as an antidiarrhoeal drug and as an adjunct to rehydration therapies.

Presentation

Loperamide is available both as a prescription medicine and as an 'over-the-counter' medication. It is commonly found in either capsule or syrup preparations. Capsules are usually of 2 mg strength and syrups of 1 mg/5 ml strength.

Occurrence of poisoning incidences

Since the launch of the VPIS in 1992, approximately 10 enquiries per annum have been made to the London centre about the ingestion by dogs of products containing loperamide. It is predominantly accidental ingestion of the 'over-the-counter' capsules in the home environment that is the cause of the poisonings, rather than accidental overdosing by owners or veterinarians.

Recommended dosage

In dogs, the recommended dose for management of diarrhoea is 0.04–0.2 mg/kg body weight orally two or three times daily. It is remarked that in dogs the drug may cause some sedative effects.

In the experience of the VPIS, doses greater than 0.1 mg/kg body weight in collie breeds might produce toxic effects.

Toxicity

Loperamide ingestions usually result in the rapid onset of mild clinical effects. Serious or fatal cases are rare. All but one of the cases reported to VPISLn have recovered without sequelae. A fatal case was reported in a 6-week-old Yorkshire Terrier puppy.

According to the literature:

- Ingestion of 0.63 mg/kg body weight can produce vomiting.
- Ingestion of 5 mg/kg body weight resulted in hind-limb paresis.

- Doses between 1.25 and 5 mg/kg body weight per day may result in more severe clinical effects including vomiting, depression, excessive salivation and weight loss.
- A dose of 5 mg/kg body weight per day produced haemorrhagic enteritis.
- The LD_{50} is quoted as 40 mg/kg body weight.
- Collie breeds may be more susceptible.

In the experience of the VPISLn:

- Doses between 0.5 and 0.8 mg/kg body weight in non-Collie breeds produced vomiting only.
- A dose of 0.12 mg/kg body weight in one Collie produced excessive salivation, inappetence and vocalising (VPISLn case 97/86921).
- A dose of 0.42 mg/kg body weight in a Collie resulted in profound sedation and unresponsiveness, bradycardia, respiratory depression, constricted pupils and hypothermia. The animal recovered with supportive care (VPISLn case 96/164267).
- A dose of 14.3 mg/kg body weight given to a 6-week-old Yorkshire Terrier by the owner resulted in collapse, coma and death (VPISLn case 97/19955).
- Collie breeds appear more susceptible.

Mechanism of toxicity

Loperamide is a weak opioid drug with potent anti-motility and anti-secretory properties. At therapeutic doses it has no CNS effects and does not cross the blood–brain barrier. It is possible that, as with Ivermectin, the blood–brain barrier of collie breeds allows significant diffusion of loperamide.

Loperamide exerts its pharmacological effects by reducing peristalsis in the lower intestine. This is achieved through increased circular contractions and decreased longitudinal contractions of the intestinal and colonic smooth muscle. This results in prolongation of intestinal transit time, allowing for greater absorption of fluid and electrolytes. The mechanism is mediated by opioid receptors and perhaps also by calcium channel blocking activity. Loperamide does not cause a delay in gastric emptying.

In high doses, the activation of opioid receptors in the CNS together with the above effects on smooth muscle contractility are responsible for the toxic effects.

Kinetics and metabolism

Loperamide is moderately well absorbed from the gastrointestinal tract. It is metabolised in the liver and the plasma half-life ranges between 6 and 14 hours.

Clinical effects

Collie breeds may be more susceptible to the effects of loperamide. Effects may occur within 30 minutes and usually within 6 hours following single acute exposures.

Vomiting, constipation, abdominal tenderness, constricted pupils, unreactive pupils, salivation, vocalisation, circling, head pressing, incoordination and ataxia (sometimes in hind limbs only) are the common effects. In more severe cases depression, haemorrhagic diarrhoea, hypothermia, bradycardia, bradypnoea, drowsiness, coma and collapse may occur.

Clinical effects may persist for 4–24 hours.

Hypersalivation, hypothermia, bradycardia, cyanosis, weight loss and haemorrhagic enteritis have been reported after prolonged administrations of doses between 1.25 and 5 mg/kg body weight per day.

Treatment

Treatment is necessary if a dose greater than 0.4 mg/kg body weight has been ingested in non-Collie breeds. In Collie breeds, treatment is advocated if 0.2 mg/kg body weight has been exceeded.

If within 2 hours of ingestion, induce vomiting (provided that the animal is not too depressed or drowsy) or perform gastric lavage.

Emetics:

(a) Xylazine	Dose:	0.2 mg/kg body weight i.v.; 0.5–1 mg/kg body weight i.m. or s.c.
(b) Ipecacuanha	Dose:	1–2 ml/kg body weight (maximum 20 ml) orally
(c) Soda crystal.		

The use of adsorbents, particularly activated charcoal, is not indicated as they may increase constipation in the animal.

Treatment is otherwise supportive. The animal may require rehydration. A minimum period of 6 hours observation is advocated.

If there is evidence of opioid-based depression (constricted pupils, drowsiness, salivation, hind-limb paresis) then naloxone should be administered.

Naloxone dose: 0.04–1 mg/kg body weight by i.v., i.m. or s.c. injection. In severe cases, repeated doses may be necessary for as long as 24 hours.

References and further reading

VPIS (London) past cases up to 97/86921.

Buronfosse F, Buronfosse T and Berny P (1998). Breed variability to loperamide susceptibility in dogs. *Veterinary and Human Toxicology* **40(3)**, 170.

Hugnet C *et al.* (1996). Loperamide poisoning in the dog. *Veterinary and Human Toxicology* **38(1)**, 31–33.

Johnson SE (1989). Loperamide: a novel antidiarrhoeal drug. *Continuing Education* **11**, 1373–1375.

Papich MG (1990). Toxicoses from over-the-counter human drugs. *Veterinary Clinics of North America: Small Animal Practice* **20(2)**, 431–451.

Staley EC and Staley EE (1994). Loperamide intoxication in a seven-week-old pup. *Veterinary and Human Toxicology* **36(5)**, 451.

Metaldehyde

Type of product

Metaldehyde is a common ingredient of molluscicide preparations.

Presentation

Usually as small blue–green coloured pellets containing about 3–8% w/w metaldehyde in a bran/wheat filler. Some products contain animal repellent components.

Liquid preparations are also available. These may contain up to 20% w/w metaldehyde. They are usually clear, colourless solutions. Some may contain ethylene glycol as an excipient.

Occurrence of poisoning incidences

Since the launch of the VPIS in 1992, between 30 and 60 enquiries about ingestion of metaldehyde containing slug bait have been handled each year. These cases predominantly involve dogs. Over 80% of these animals have presented to a surgery displaying clinical effects. Fatal outcomes with this agent are more common than any other according to the VPIS London data. Between 10 and 23% of the cases referred have a fatal outcome.

Toxicity

Metaldehyde, which is most commonly ingested by dogs in the form of slug pellets, is toxic to dogs. Slug pellets appear to be quite attractive to dogs. It frequently results in prolonged convulsant activity. Fatalities due to respiratory failure frequently result.

According to the literature:

- Quoted LD_{50} values for dogs cover a wide range, the lowest reported value being 60 mg/kg body weight.
- Assuming a fatal dose in dogs for metaldehyde of 60 mg/kg body weight and a bait of 8% w/w strength, then the fatal dose in dogs would be 750 mg bait/kg body weight of the animal.
- Clinical effects have been reported following ingestion of total doses of 200 g of pellets (Rose).
- Smaller dogs tend to have higher mortality than larger ones.

In the experience of the VPISLn:

- Fatalities have been reported following ingestion of 250 g of bait (VPISLn case 85/7443).

- A 35 kg Retriever consumed a maximum of 500 g of bait. Within 2 hours the animal was twitching, tachycardic, tachypnoeic and hyperthermic. Intravenous saline was given, with diazepam and pentobarbitone sedation/anaesthesia and calcium supplementation. The animal deteriorated and was euthanased (VPISLn case 94/47627).
- A 30 kg Great Dane ingested 400 g of slug pellets. Within 30 minutes the animal had salivation, convulsions, total collapse and, despite i.v. fluids, pentobarbitone and diazepam, died within 3 hours (VPISLn case 94/54462).
- A 5-year-old Collie ate a maximum quantity of 500 g of slug pellets. Within 30 minutes the animal had hyperaesthesia, collapse, tremors and hyperthermia. The animal was given an emetic, i.v. fluid support with Hartmann's solution, and maintained under pentobarbitone anaesthesia for 12 hours. On cessation of anaesthetic the animal gradually recovered, with mild convulsant episodes being successfully controlled with diazepam (VPISLn case 94/74663).

Mechanism of toxicity

The mechanism of metaldehyde toxicity is not clearly understood. It is most frequently suggested that the primary toxic agent is acetaldehyde, which would be formed if ingested metaldehyde were hydrolysed by gastric acid. The suggestion is that the subsequent metabolism of acetaldehyde to carbon dioxide is a slower reaction than the hydrolysis one resulting in acetaldehyde formation, and that acetaldehyde levels therefore rise, causing the clinical effects. There is, however, no *in vivo* evidence for this process or mechanism. Indeed, it has been shown that in the cases of both paraldehyde and ethanol the conversion of acetaldehyde to carbon dioxide occurs at a rate faster than the acetaldehyde formation from the parent compound.

Recent work has demonstrated that other factors may be involved. In mice metaldehyde exposure has been linked to a decrease in the levels of the inhibitory neurotransmitter gamma-aminobutyric acid (GABA), noradrenaline and 5-HT, as well as causing an increase in monoamine oxidase (MAO) activity. Mortality correlated well with decrease in GABA activity and it is suggested that the impairment of GABA inhibitory activity may be causative of the convulsant activity seen in metaldehyde exposures. The exact mechanism is therefore unknown and it seems unlikely that acetaldehyde can be the sole cause of toxic effects.

Kinetics and metabolism

Metaldehyde is reportedly rapidly absorbed from the gastrointestinal tract and metabolised to acetaldehyde. This is further metabolised to carbon dioxide or excreted in urine.

Clinical effects

Onset may be very rapid, often within 30 minutes of ingestion, but may be delayed for up to 3 hours.

Incoordination, irritability, anxiety, hyperpnoea and tachycardia are reported. Congested and pale mucous membranes, hypersalivation, dilated pupils, nystagmus, hyperthermia, dehydration, vomiting, haematemesis, diarrhoea (may be green in colour if ingested product was dyed), borborygmi, abdominal tenderness, and ataxia are all documented. Occasionally, animals become drowsy.

The classic clinical presentation is that of hyperaesthesia, muscle spasm, twitching and tremors, leading to opisthotonus and continuous convulsions. These may have a duration of 24 hours or more. In serious cases this may lead to collapse, loss of consciousness, dyspnoea, respiratory depression and cyanosis. Deaths are usually due to respiratory failure. Atrial fibrillation has been reported in VPISLn case 93/79105.

Liver damage is a secondary effect and has caused fatalities 2–3 days post-exposure. Renal damage has been reported in other species.

Long-term sequelae are reported. These include diarrhoea, apparent memory loss and temporary blindness, which resolved within 3 weeks.

Post-mortem findings

Findings include hyperaemia of the liver and kidneys, degeneration of liver cells and of ganglion cells in the brain. Petechial and ecchymotic haemorrhages in the gastrointestinal mucosa are documented. Hyperaemia and interstitial haemorrhages in the lung are reported. Massive subendocardial and subepicardial haemorrhages have also been seen.

Treatment

Treatment is advised for ingestion of any quantity of metaldehyde by a dog.

If the dog is presented to the surgery within 2 hours *and* is asymptomatic then vomiting can be safely induced. Alternatively, gastric lavage may be considered. Metaldehyde reportedly does not bind to activated charcoal and therefore use of adsorbents is not indicated.

Emetics:

(a)	Apomorphine	Dose:	0.05 mg/kg body weight i.v. or i.m.; 0.1 mg/kg body weight s.c.
(b)	Xylazine	Dose:	0.2 mg/kg body weight i.v.; 0.5–1 mg/kg body weight i.m. or s.c.
(c)	Ipecacuanha	Dose:	1–2 ml/kg body weight (maximum 20 ml) orally
(d)	Soda crystal.		

All dogs require observation for a minimum of 4 hours.

If the animal is or becomes symptomatic then it is advisable to anaesthetise or sedate the dog to control convulsant activity and to allow gastric lavage to be performed if appropriate.

Many authors have advised keeping the dog sedated but still slightly hyperaesthetic and in control of their vital reflexes until the clinical effects are seen to resolve, and then allowing them to slowly recover. Continued sedation has been necessary for well over 24 hours in some cases.

Others, particularly in cases that present with severe signs, have advocated deep anaesthesia for 24–48 hours, then allowing recovery of consciousness, with a return to anaesthesia if clinical effects reappear. During this time body fluids need to be maintained by alternating lactated Ringers and dextrose saline drips.

Drugs used to achieve these procedures in past cases and reports have included diazepam, pentobarbitone and acepromazine. Cases where the latter have been used reportedly required far less supervision.

Doses recommended:

(a) Diazepam	0.5 mg/kg body weight i.v. repeated every 10 minutes up to three times if needed.	
(b) Acepromazine	1–3 mg/kg body weight orally; 0.03–0.1 mg/kg body weight i.m., or s.c.; 0.03 mg/kg body weight by slow i.v. injection. (In some past cases doses as high as 16.5 mg/kg body weight have been given over a 45-min period with good result.)	
(c) Pentobarbitone	25–30 mg/kg by slow intravenous infusion.	

To prevent development of pulmonary oedema, it is advisable to turn the dog every couple of hours.

Lactated Ringers solution has been recommended for animals that are acidotic and/or dehydrated. Parenteral administration of dextrose saline or calcium borogluconate has been suggested to prevent liver damage.

Both vitamins and antibiotics have been given in many past cases.

References and further reading

VPIS (London) past cases up to 97/118197.

Bishop CHG (1975). Blindness associated with metaldehyde poisoning. *Veterinary Record* **96(19)**, 438.

Blaine DR (1977). Treatment of metaldehyde poisoning in dogs. *Veterinary Medicine/ Small Animal Clinician* **72(6)**, 1009–1011.

Booze TF and Oehme FW (1985). Metaldehyde toxicity: a review. *Veterinary and Human Toxicology* **27(1)**, 11–19.

Cruikshank AK (1982). Metaldehyde and paraquat poisoning. *Veterinary Record* **111(7)**, 149–150.

Mayer S (1991). Poison – metaldehyde. *In Practice* **13(2)**, 57.

Oehme FW (1987). Clinical toxicology in small animals. In *Veterinary Clinical Toxicology, Proceedings No. 103* (Proceedings of a conference held at the University of Sydney, Australia, 24–28 August, 1987), pp. 443–447.

Rose IRB (1986). Anaesthetic control for metaldehyde poisoning. *Veterinary Record* **119(15)**, 388.

Turner T (1967). Metaldehyde poisoning in the dog. *Veterinary Record* **80(4)**, 184.

Turner T (1973). Toxicity of metaldehyde to dogs. *Veterinary Record* **93(19)**, 524.

Udall ND (1973). The toxicity of the molluscicides metaldehyde and methiocarb to dogs. *Veterinary Record* **93**, 420–422.

Von Berg R and Stout T (1991). Toxicology update – metaldehyde. *Journal of Applied Toxicology* **11 (5)**, 377–378.

Webster CJ and Webster JM (1986). Anaesthetic control for metaldehyde poisoning. *Veterinary Record* **119(20)**, 511–512.

Methiocarb

Type of product

Carbamate pesticide used principally as a molluscicide.

Presentation

Commonly available as blue coloured pellets containing 4% methiocarb. Some molluscicide preparations may contain a combination of methiocarb and metaldehyde (see the chapter on metaldehyde).

Occurrence of poisoning incidences

Since its launch, the VPIS London centre has received a small number of enquiries about methiocarb exposures in dogs. These enquiries represent approximately 0.25% of the total enquiries. In all but two cases the animals have exhibited clinical effects. Several fatal outcomes have been reported.

Toxicity

According to the literature:

- The LD_{50} of methiocarb in dogs is 25 mg/kg body weight.
- Assuming a fatal dose of 25 mg/kg body weight and a bait of 4% w/w strength, a fatal dose is calculated as 625 mg bait/kg body weight in dogs.

In the experience of VPISLn:

Several fatal cases have been reported. Clinical effects in these cases have been those anticipated. In one case death occurred within 2 hours. At post-mortem the stomach was found to be full of pellets (VPISLn case 94/41428).

Mechanism of toxicity

Like organophosphates, carbamates bind to and inhibit acetylcholinesterase. This results in accumulation of the neurotransmitter acetylcholine and activation of nicotinic receptors at skeletal muscle end plates, autonomic ganglia and within the CNS, and of muscarinic receptors at smooth muscle myoneural junctions and exocrine and endocrine secretory systems. Therefore both nicotinic and muscarinic effects occur, although nicotinic receptors rapidly become desensitised. Myopathy is thought to be secondary to excessive acetylcholine stimulation of muscle.

Compared with the phosphorylated enzyme that results from organophosphate poisoning, the carbamylated acetylcholinesterase is more unstable, and spontaneous reversal to the carbamate and acetylcholinesterase occurs. As a result, the effects resulting from carbamate poisoning tend to be of much shorter duration compared with those of organophosphate poisoning and use of cholinesterase reactivators (such as pralidoxime) is unnecessary. Atropine acts as a non-competitive antagonist by blocking the effect of the muscarinic receptors on target organs.

Kinetics and metabolism

Carbamates may be absorbed from the gastrointestinal tract, through the skin and following exposure to high concentrations via the lungs. They are rapidly excreted.

Clinical effects

Onset of effects is usually between 30 minutes and 3 hours. Recovery may take 1–2 days because of the slow-release nature of the pellets.

Mild to moderate effects normally include salivation, bronchial hypersecretion, ataxia, diarrhoea, constricted pupils, muscle fasciculation, tremors and twitching, weakness, shaking, hyperaesthesia, pyrexia, restlessness and urinary incontinence.

In severe cases collapse, bradycardia, respiratory depression, convulsions, cyanosis and coma may occur.

Myopathy occurs rarely following recovery.

Carbamates do not cause the delayed neurotoxicity sometimes observed with organophosphate insecticides. This is due to the lack of ageing with carbamates.

Laboratory findings

These are generally non-specific and include increased packed cell volume (PCV), raised serum aspartate transaminase (AST) and creatinine phosphokinase (CPK). Elevated serum amylase may be noted.

Post-mortem findings

There are no characteristic lesions observed in carbamate insecticide poisoned animals. Pulmonary changes may be observed including bronchoconstriction, increased bronchial secretions and pulmonary oedema. Pancreatitis may be present.

Treatment

If more than the equivalent of 10 mg/kg body weight of methiocarb has been ingested within 2 hours, induce vomiting or perform gastric lavage, and then administer adsorbents.

Emetics:

(a)	Apomorphine	Dose:	0.05 mg/kg body weight i.v. or i.m.; 0.1 mg/kg body weight s.c.
(b)	Xylazine	Dose:	0.2 mg/kg body weight i.v.; 0.5–1 mg/kg body weight i.m. or s.c.
(c)	Ipecacuanha	Dose:	1–2 ml/kg body weight (maximum 20 ml) orally
(d)	Soda crystal.		

Adsorbents:

(a)	Activated charcoal	Dose:	2 g/kg body weight orally
(b)	BCK granules®	Dose:	6–18 g orally two or three times daily.

Further management is largely symptomatic; in particular body temperature should be maintained, and blood gases and electrolytes monitored and corrected. Rehydration may be required.

If sedation is required then diazepam may be given. Dose: 0.5 mg/kg body weight i.v. repeated every 10 minutes up to three times if needed.

Atropine should be given to reverse cholinergic effects. Dose: 0.2–2 mg/kg body weight (one-quarter of the dose given i.v. and the remainder s.c. or i.m.) repeated as required (usually every 45–90 minutes, initially). Large doses may be required for effect.

Atropine has no effect on nicotinic receptors and will not counteract skeletal muscle tremors, weakness or neuromuscular paralysis. However, effects from carbamates such as methiocarb are generally short-lived and cholinesterase reactivators such as pralidoxime are not required.

Contra-indicated drugs

Phenothiazine sedatives and succinylcholine should be avoided because of the neuromuscular blocking activity, since they will exacerbate the toxicity of methiocarb. Antibiotics such as aminoglycosides (e.g. streptomycin, gentamicin, neomycin, kanamycin), polypeptides (e.g. polymixin A and B) and clindamycin should also be avoided, since they may have neuromuscular blocking effects. Benzodiazepines, opioids and barbiturates should be used cautiously because of their CNS depressant effects.

Laboratory investigations

Cholinesterase activity determination may be considered. It is advised that whole blood from unaffected animals should also be submitted as a control. Although not a uniformly reliable indicator, a decrease of 50% or more of normal activity generally indicates significant inhibition and in many cases the cholinesterase activity is less than 25% of normal. In cases of carbamate poisoning, whole blood samples must be rapidly collected, frozen and transported to the laboratory because of spontaneous reactivation of cholinesterase.

References and further reading

VPIS (London) past cases up to 97/91797.

Fikes JD (1990). Organophosphate and carbamate insecticides. *Veterinary Clinics of North America: Small Animal Practice* **20(2)**, 353–367.

McEntree K *et al.* (1994). Acute polymyopathy after carbamate poisoning in a dog. *Veterinary Record* **134**, 88–89.

Udall ND (1973). The toxicity of the molluscicides metaldehyde and methiocarb to dogs. *Veterinary Record* **93**, 420–421.

Mistletoe / *Viscum album*

The plant

Viscum album (common name, mistletoe) belongs to the Viscaceae family, though was formerly classified in the Loranthaceae family.

The plant grows, as a partial parasite, on deciduous trees. It has a woody appearance with long stems that bear thick, dark-green leaves of 5–8 cm in length. The plant flowers in spring with clusters of yellowish flowers. Fruits remain on the plant throughout winter. They are characteristic white, semi-translucent berries containing a viscous juice and a single dark-coloured seed.

Occurrence of poisoning incidences

Since the launch of the VPIS, the centre in London has received a small number of enquiries each year regarding ingestion of mistletoe by dogs. These usually occur at Christmas time when plant parts being used as festive decoration are found indoors. Over 70% of these cases remained asymptomatic. Those with clinical effects displayed mild gastrointestinal effects only.

Toxicity

The plant is considered by the VPIS to be of low toxicity. It is possible that some reports are confusing the effects of the American mistletoe (Phoradendron) as those of *Viscum album*.

According to the literature:

- Ingestion of a spray of mistletoe with berries resulted in the development of neurological signs with ataxia, incoordination, head nodding and hyperaesthesia. The dog became hypothermic and died some 50 hours post ingestion.

In the experience of the VPISLn:

- Two Jack Russell terriers ate 10 mistletoe berries between them. They both vomited and showed generalised weakness. Both recovered with supportive care and rehydration (VPISLn case 93/130002).

Mechanism of toxicity

The berries, leaves and stems of the plant are all potentially toxic. They contain lectins and viscotoxins, which are both protein structures.

Experimentally, lectins are found to inhibit protein synthesis and cell growth

Clinical effects

Vomiting, diarrhoea, salivation, and weakness are the only effects reported in past VPIS cases. These effects have generally been rapid in onset.

The literature describes cases where effects have been delayed for several hours and where ataxia, constricting pupils, hyperaesthesia, polyuria and hypotension have been reported. CNS effects are also detailed in some reports including convulsions, hyperactivity, drowsiness or coma, and respiratory distress.

Treatment

Gastric decontamination using gastric lavage, emesis or adsorbents is not necessary unless huge amounts of plant material have been ingested.

Where vomiting is profuse, use of anti-emetics such as metoclopramide may be considered.

Metoclopramide dose: 0.5–1 mg/kg body weight orally, s.c. or i.m. every 6–8 hours; 1–2 mg/kg body weight per day by slow i.v. infusion.

Management should otherwise be supportive, particularly ensuring that the animal is well hydrated.

In the unlikely event of hyperaesthesia or convulsions occurring, diazepam may be given. Diazepam dose: 0.5 mg/kg body weight i.v. repeated every 10 minutes up to three times if needed.

References and Further reading

VPIS (London) past cases up to 97/189127.

Greatorex JC (1966). Some unusual cases of plant poisoning in animals. *Veterinary Record* **78**, 725–727.

Naproxen

Type of product

Naproxen is a non-steroidal anti-inflammatory drug (NSAID).

Presentation

Naproxen is available in the UK as a prescription medicine with indications for use in management of pain and inflammation in rheumatic diseases, gout and dysmenorrhoea. It is sold under various brand names in tablet, liquid suspension and suppository preparations.

The dose of naproxen in tablet preparations is variable, but usually 250 mg, 275 mg and 500 mg.

Some preparations are modified release. Liquid suspensions are commonly of 125 mg/5 ml strength, and suppositories of 500 mg.

A dose of 275 mg of naproxen sodium is equivalent to 250 mg of naproxen. Some preparations, such as Napratec®, have tablets of misoprostol designed to be taken simultaneously.

Occurrence of poisoning incidences

Ingestions of naproxen by companion animals feature regularly in the enquiries made to the VPIS London centre. Since 1993, between five and 10 enquiries per year have been received, with almost all cases occurring in dogs.

Recommended dosage

In dogs the recommended dose is 5 mg/kg body weight initially and then 2 mg/kg body weight daily for management of inflammation and pain.

Toxicity

Dogs are particularly sensitive to the propionic acid group of NSAIDs, which includes naproxen. In particular, they are prone to develop severe gastric ulceration and intestinal irritation. In the case of naproxen the toxicity appears to be lower than some of the other drugs in the group such as ibuprofen and flurbiprofen. Although there have been no post-mortem studies in the literature to confirm the presence of gastric ulceration and intestinal inflammation in naproxen cases, the clinical effects reported are consistent with such findings. Gastroscopy has revealed ulceration in the pyloric region of the stomach in one case in the literature.

According to the literature:

- LD_{50} quoted as 1 g/kg body weight.
- A 2-month-old pug given a total of 110 mg/kg body weight naproxen over 4 days exhibited depression, melena, lethargy vomiting and anaemia. The animal survived with treatment, which included blood transfusions and gastroprotective medications.
- A dog given 125 mg twice daily for five days and developed depression, weakness, tar-like faeces, anorexia, vomiting and anaemia. Following intensive management with transfusions the animal recovered.

In the experience of the VPISLn:

- No effects were seen in a dog given 11 mg/kg body weight acutely.
- One dog received a dose of 375 mg/kg body weight and developed no clinical effects. The animal had been given an emetic shortly after ingestion (VPISLn case 96/52958).
- An acute dosing of 40 mg/kg body weight produced vomiting, melena, diarrhoea and dehydration in a Dalmatian. The dog survived with treatment (VPISLn case 95/68608).
- Doses as high as 283 and 588 mg/kg body weight have been survived by dogs, though both developed severe gastrointestinal distress, melena and vomiting. Both received supportive care with use of cimetidine (VPISLn cases 94/26705 and 94/ 89197).

Mechanism of toxicity

Like other propionic acid-derived NSAIDs, naproxen competitively inhibits the cyclo-oxygenase step of prostaglandin synthesis. Such inhibition and subsequent reduction in levels of PGI_2 and PGE_2 can account for the major effects seen in poisoning cases.

In the gastrointestinal tract prostaglandins have a cytoprotective function, as they control production of gastric acid, stimulate secretion of mucous and bicarbonate by the gastric epithelium and maintain mucosal blood flow by causing vasodilatation. Deficiency will result in increased gastric acid secretion and reduction in mucous production and mucosal blood flow. These effects and the acidic nature of the drug itself all increase risk of ulcer formation.

In the kidneys, prostaglandins maintain afferent arteriolar dilatation, regulating renal blood flow and glomerular filtration rate. They also have a role in control of renin release and maintenance of water balance. NSAID inhibition of prostaglandin synthesis will result in reduction of renal blood flow and disrupt normal renal function and homeostatic mechanisms. Constriction of renal arterioles may result in renal papillary necrosis. These effects may be more evident in animals that are dehydrated or volume depleted.

Kinetics and metabolism

Naproxen is rapidly absorbed upon ingestion by dogs. Peak plasma concentrations usually occur between 0.5 and 3 hours post-ingestion. The drug is largely bound to serum proteins on absorption and has a low volume of distribution. Faecal elimination is the primary route of excretion and the plasma half-life is quoted as 35 hours or more (values in a range 51–75 hours are quoted in some references).

Clinical effects

The initial clinical effects following acute exposures usually occur within 8 hours. With more prolonged dosing, effects may be delayed for 4 days or more.

Clinical effects include vomiting (often persistent), haematemesis, diarrhoea, melena, abdominal tenderness and anorexia. Mucous membranes may be pale or congested. Weakness, ataxia, incoordination, lethargy, collapse, dehydration, depression and drowsiness have been noted.

Dyspnoea, hyperventilation, tachycardia, vocalising, agitation, hyperactivity, hyperaesthesia, tremors, twitching or convulsions have been reported following ingestion of other drugs of the same group and could be anticipated for naproxen ingestion.

Evidence of gastrointestinal irritation and renal impairment is to be expected from 12–24 hours after ingestion. Compared to the effects seen with other NSAIDs, anaemia appears more common with naproxen exposures. There may be protracted vomiting, pyrexia, anorexia, polyuria, polydipsia, dehydration and collapse.

Renal impairment should be anticipated if large doses (greater than 150 mg/kg body weight) have been ingested. This would be characterised by oliguria, azotemia, and elevated creatinine and BUN. Renal failure can theoretically occur and may be delayed. Hypotensive or dehydrated animals are potentially at greater risk from renal effects, as are those with pre-existing renal impairment.

Post-mortem findings

There may be evidence of gastrointestinal congestion and/or haemorrhage, gastric ulceration or perforation and renal tubule papillary necrosis.

Treatment

Treatment is advocated if a dose of 10 mg/kg body weight has been exceeded (5 mg/kg body weight in animals that are dehydrated, hypotensive or have pre-existing renal insufficiency).

If within 3 hours of ingestion, induce vomiting or perform gastric lavage and then administer adsorbents.

Emetics:

(a) Apomorphine	Dose:	0.05 mg/kg body weight i.v. or i.m.; 0.1 mg/kg body weight s.c.
(b) Xylazine	Dose:	0.2 mg/kg body weight i.v.; 0.5–1 mg/kg body weight i.m. or s.c.
(c) Ipecacuanha	Dose:	1–2 ml/kg body weight (maximum 20 ml) orally

(d) Soda crystal.

Adsorbents:

(a) Activated charcoal	Dose:	2 g/kg body weight orally
(b) BCK granules®	Dose:	6–18g orally two or three times daily

If there is severe or persistent vomiting then anti-emetics should be administered. If adsorbents have been administered this may reduce efficacy of orally administered anti-emetics. In such cases, parenteral administration is preferable. Either metoclopramide or acepromazine may be used; the latter has a longer duration of action.

(a) Metoclopramide	Dose:	0.5–1 mg/kg body weight orally, s.c. or i.m. every 6–8 hours; 1–2 mg/kg body weight per day by slow i.v. infusion
(b) Acepromazine	Dose:	0.03–0.1 mg/kg body weight i.v., i.m., or s.c. (use lower dose if giving i.v.); 1–3 mg/kg body weight orally.

Gastric effects

In *all* cases where treatment has been necessary, the animals should be administered ulcer-healing or ulcer-preventing drugs.

The H_2-receptor blocking drugs cimetidine, ranitidine and famotidine reduce gastric acid and pepsin secretions, reducing the risk of ulcer formation and allowing ulcers to heal. Omeprazole inhibits the proton pump responsible for gastric acid production by the parietal cells. It is more potent and has a longer duration of action (greater than 24 hours) than the three aforementioned H_2-receptor blockers and its use should be reserved for animals who are not responding to other therapies.

Sucralfate is an ulcer-coating agent that binds to proteins at an ulcer site, protecting it from further gastric acid and pepsin attack.

Misoprostol is a synthetic prostaglandin analogue that in effect replaces the prostaglandins whose production is inhibited by naproxen. Administration shortly after naproxen ingestion will therefore ensure continued control of gastric acid secretion and increased mucous production, thereby preventing ulcer formation. Its use is contraindicated in animals who have already developed ulcers following NSAID ingestion.

Suggested regimen

The following treatment protocol is recommended for a 14-day period.

Either

Cimetidine   Dose: 5–10 mg/kg body weight i.v., i.m. or
                orally every 6–8 hours

Notes

1. If absorbents have been administered then parenteral routes should be employed in the initial stages to minimise binding to drug.
2. If the i.v. route is to be used then administer by slow i.v. infusion over 30 minutes to reduce risk of hypotension and arrhythmias.
3. If metoclopramide has been used or sucralfate is to be used then a period of 2 hours should elapse before cimetidine is administered.
4. Adverse effect – cimetidine blocks liver microsomal enzymes and therefore hepatic drug metabolism.

Or

Ranitidine   Dose: 0.5–4 mg/kg body weight i.v., s.c. or
                orally every 12 hours.

Notes

1. If adsorbents have been administered then parenteral routes should be employed in the initial stages to minimise binding to drug.
2. If metoclopramide has been used or sucralfate is to be used then a period of 2 hours should elapse before ranitidine is administered.

Or

Famotidine   Dose: 500 μg/kg body weight orally every 12 hours.

Notes

1. Where adsorbents have been administered, a period of 2 hours should elapse before famotidine is administered to minimise binding to drug.
2. If sucralfate is to be used then a period of 2 hours should elapse before famotidine is administered.

Where ingestion was recent and >10 mg/kg body weight of naproxen may have been ingested, also give:

Misoprostol   Dose: 1–5 μg/kg body weight orally every 6–8 hours for 24 hours.

Notes

1. Where adsorbents have been administered, a period of 2 hours should elapse before misoprostol is administered to minimise binding to drug.
2. If ulceration is already suspected or confirmed, misoprostol should not be given and sucralfate given instead.

3. Adverse effects – misoprostol may cause vomiting, diarrhoea and abdominal tenderness and abortions in pregnant animals.

Where >10 mg/kg body weight naproxen may have been ingested and ulceration is either suspected or confirmed, give:

Sucralfate   Dose: in dogs <20 kg body weight 500 mg/dog orally every 6–8 hours; in dogs >20kg body weight 1 g/dog orally every 6–8 hours.

Notes

1. Where adsorbents have been administered, a period of 2 hours should elapse before sucralfate is administered to minimise binding to drug.
2. If cimetidine, ranitidine or famotidine are to be used then sucralfate should be given 2 hours beforehand as it requires an acid environment for maximum efficacy.
3. Ideally, sucralfate should be administered on an empty stomach, at least 1 hour prior to food.

If the animal does not respond to the above therapies then administration of omeprazole may be considered. The recommended dose is 0.5–1.5 mg/kg body weight orally every 24 hours.

Other care

Management is otherwise largely symptomatic and supportive. Ensure adequate hydration and good urine output. In some cases, dopamine may be necessary to increase renal perfusion and to minimise renal insufficiency (dose: 1–3 μg/kg body weight per minute as constant i.v. infusion).

Following large naproxen ingestions, dogs appear particularly prone to anaemia. In some cases, blood transfusion has been required. If possible blood gases and electrolytes should be checked and corrected, especially if there is evidence of renal dysfunction and/or oliguria. Bicarbonate should be given to correct acidosis if present. *Caution* – dopamine precipitates in bicarbonate solutions, so these fluids should not be administered together. If the animal is hyperkalaemic, then this should be corrected using dextrose (dose: 20% solution given 1 ml/kg body weight i.v.) together with insulin if available (dose: 0.5 units/kg body weight).

Diazepam may be given if there is any convulsant activity (dose: 0.5 mg/kg body weight i.v. repeated every 10 minutes up to three times if needed).

Bland diets are recommended.

Enhanced elimination

Naproxen is largely protein-bound and extensively metabolised and therefore alkaline diuresis or urine alkalinisation, dialysis or haemoperfusion are unlikely to enhance elimination.

Investigative

Blood naproxen levels are not helpful in management except as confirmation of ingestion. Interpretation of levels is difficult and case management is better based on clinical condition of the animal. In any event, such analysis is not routinely offered by many laboratories.

Blood counts should be instituted for cases with clinical effects.

In severe cases, radiography or gastroscopy may be employed to assess gastric mucosal damage.

Increases in prothrombin time or INR are rarely reported in naproxen overdoses.

References

VPIS (London) past cases up to 97/02428.

Dye TL (1997). Naproxen toxicosis in a puppy. *Veterinary and Human Toxicology* **39(3)**, 157–159.

Elliott GA (1988). The propionic acids. Gastrointestinal toxicity in various species. *Toxicologic Pathology* **16(2)**, 245–250.

Frey HH and Rich B (1981). Pharmacokinetics of naproxen in the dog. *American Journal of Veterinary Research* **42**, 1615–1617.

Gilmour MA and Walshaw R (1987). Naproxen induced toxicosis in a dog. *Journal of the American Veterinary Medical Association* **191(11)**, 1431–1432.

Jones RD et al. (1992). Non-steroidal anti-inflammatory drug toxicosis in dogs and cats: 240 cases. *Journal of the American Veterinary Medical Association* **201(3)**, 475–478.

Kore AM (1990). Toxicology of non-steroidal anti-inflammatory drugs. *Veterinary Clinics of North America: Small Animal Practice* **20**, 419–429.

Kore AM (1997). Over-the-counter analgesic drug toxicoses in small animals. *Veterinary Medicine* **92 (2)**, 158–165.

Lascelles D and Balmer T (1997). Are all NSAIDs the same? *Veterinary Times* **24(4)**, 34–37.

Roudebush P and Morse GE (1981). Naproxen toxicosis in a dog. *Journal of the American Veterinary Medical Association* **179(8)**, 805–806.

Smith RE (1982). Naproxen toxicosis. *Journal of the American Veterinary Medical Association* **180(2)**, 107.

Vollmar AM (1993). Clinico-toxicologic aspects of non-steroidal anti-inflammatory agents in the dog and cat. *Tierarztliche Praxis* **21(2)**, 149–152 (in German).

Zech R et al. (1993). Plasma and tissue kinetics of phenylbutazone and naproxen in dogs. *Archives Internationale de Pharmacodynamie et de Therapie* **325**, 113–128.

Organophosphate insecticides

Type of product

Organophosphate insecticides are widely used as garden and household pesticides, as well as in agriculture.

Presentation

Formulations include liquids, sprays and powders, which may be used as supplied or diluted; liquid preparations often contain organic solvents. In veterinary medicine, they are found in sheep-dips, and pedicullicide lotions. Shampoos, aqueous and alcoholic lotions are also used as human pedicullicides and scabicides. They are also used in flea collars.

Substances included are **chlorfenvinphos, chlorpyrifos, demeton-*S*-methyl, diazinon, dichlorvos, dimethoate, fenthion, fenitrothion, heptenophos, malathion and pirimiphos-methyl.**

Occurrence of poisoning incidences

Since 1992, the VPIS has received an increasing percentage of enquiries about organophosphate insecticide exposures in both cats and dogs. Calls concerning these agents represent between 1.3 and 2.4% of the total enquiry load. In the early years, enquiries about pirimphos-methyl and dichlorvos containing agents predominated, although in recent years there has been a noticeable rise in enquiries concerning chlorpyrifos and diazinon as products for home use containing these active ingredients have become available.

Toxicity

Toxic doses for many of the organophosphates in dogs have not been established.

According to the literature:

Chlorfenvinphos

- The oral LD_{50} for dogs are quoted in the range greater than 1200–5000 mg/kg body weight.

Chlorpyrifos

- No oral LD_{50} is quoted for dogs.

- Dogs fed 3 mg/kg body weight daily for 2 years displayed no clinically important effects.

Demeton-S-methyl

- No oral LD_{50} for dogs is quoted.
- Dogs fed 0.036 mg/kg body weight daily for 1 year developed no clinically important effects.

Diazinon

- No oral LD_{50} for dogs is quoted.
- Dogs fed 0.02 mg/kg body weight daily for 13 weeks developed no toxic effects.

Dichlorvos

- The oral LD_{50} for dogs is quoted as 100 mg/kg body weight.
- 100 mg/kg caused respiratory failure 1–3 minutes after ingestion in 1-year-old 20 kg dogs.

Dimethoate

- The oral LD_{50} for dogs is quoted as 400 mg/kg body weight.

Fenthion

- No oral LD_{50} for dogs is quoted.

Fenitrothion

- The oral LD_{50} for dogs is quoted as greater than 681 mg/kg body weight.

Heptenophos

- The oral LD_{50} for dogs is quoted as greater than 500 mg/kg body weight

Malathion

- No oral LD_{50} for dogs is quoted.

Pirimphos-methyl

- No oral LD_{50} for dogs is quoted.
- Dogs fed 10 mg/kg body weight per day in gelatine capsules for 2 years suffered 25% mortality.
- Dogs fed 0.5 mg/kg body weight per day for 2 years showed no clinical effects.

In the experience of VPISLn:

Chlorpyrifos

- There are many cases on file of dogs ingesting chlorpyrifos, found as the active constituent of some commercially available ant baits. Very few cases develop clinical effects – in those that do, lethargy and polydipsia seem the predominant effects. No fatal cases are documented.

Demeton-S-methyl

- There are several records of demeton-S-methyl exposures on the VPIS files but none with fatal outcomes. In the documented cases, salivation and lethargy are the common effects.

Diazinon

- Many cases of diazinon exposures are on the VPIS files, including five fatal cases. Two of the fatalities had consumed flea collars containing diazinon (VPISLn cases 85/15901 and 92/44680). Two other fatal cases occurred as a result of dermal application of an incorrectly formulated insecticide product (VPISLn cases 97/65471 and 97/124773). Predominant clinical effects include tachycardia, salivation, hyperthermia, ataxia, muscle spasms, convulsions and respiratory distress.

Pirimphos-methyl

- Pirimphos-methyl exposures in dogs are also quite commonly found in VPIS cases. Ant killers appear to be the common agent ingested. Clinical effects are as anticipated – salivation, depression, tachycardia, twitching or fitting and respiratory distress. One fatal case is reported; the cause of death was respiratory arrest (VPISLn case 92/43025).

Mechanism of toxicity

Organophosphates bind to and inhibit acetylcholinesterase, resulting in accumulation of the neurotransmitter acetylcholine and activation of nicotinic receptors at skeletal muscle end plates, autonomic ganglia and within the CNS, and of muscarinic receptors at smooth muscle myoneural junctions and exocrine and endocrine secretory systems. This results in both nicotinic and muscarinic effects, although nicotinic receptors rapidly become desensitised. Myopathy is thought to be secondary to excessive acetylcholine stimulation of muscle.

Atropine acts as a non-competitive antagonist by blocking the effect of the muscarinic receptors on target organs. Pralidoxime is a cholinesterase reactivator, which dephosphorylates acetyl-cholinesterase. It is most effective when used as an adjunct to atropine therapy, as the latter is necessary to reverse the effects of muscarinic over-stimulation. Hence, animals should be atropinised before receiving it. If administered soon after acetylcholinesterase inhibition, reactivation of the enzyme will be almost complete. The treatment becomes less effective with time, as an increasing proportion of the enzyme becomes irreversibly inhibited or 'aged'.

The onset, severity and duration of poisoning are determined by the degree and route of exposure, the lipid solubility and rate of metabolism, whether transformation in the liver is required before the compound is active and whether it reversibly or irreversibly binds to cholinesterase. Some organophosphate insecticides may accumulate in adipose tissue and this may act as a source of continued exposure long after the initial contact has been terminated. In such cases, prolonged treatment may be required.

Kinetics and metabolism

Organophosphates may be absorbed from the gastrointestinal tract, through the skin and following exposure to high concentrations via the lungs. Organophosphate insecticides are metabolised in the liver principally by oxidation, hydrolysis by esterase and by transfer of portions to glutathione. Oxidation of organophosphate insecticides may result in more or less toxic products. Most organophosphates are rapidly excreted but chlorinated organophosphates (e.g. chlorpyrifos) are more lipid soluble and persist longer in tissue.

Clinical effects

Onset usually occurs within 12–24 hours. Duration may be long (several days or even weeks). Note that the organophosphate insecticide in flea collars is in a slow-release formulation and effects may be prolonged.

Clinical effects are salivation, ataxia, diarrhoea, constricted pupils, muscle fasciculation, tremors and twitching, weakness, shaking, hyperaesthesia, pyrexia, restlessness and urinary incontinence.

In severe cases, bradycardia, respiratory depression, convulsions and coma may occur.

Some organophosphate insecticides may cause delayed neurotoxicity. The organophosphate-induced delayed neuropathy (OPIDN) usually appears 2–3 weeks after the acute phase of poisoning and is thought to be due to inhibition of a poorly characterised esterase termed neuropathy target esterase (NTE). There is distal axonopathy, with progressive hind-limb weakness and ataxia. There may be paralysis, which may also involve the fore-limbs. Histological examination is characterised by symmetrical, distal, primary axonal degeneration in the central and peripheral nervous system, with secondary myelin degeneration.

Myopathy occurs rarely following recovery.

Laboratory findings

Laboratory analyses: these are generally non-specific and include increased packed cell volume (PCV), raised serum aspartate transaminase (AST) and creatinine phosphokinase (CPK). Elevated serum amylase may be noted.

Post-mortem findings

Post-mortem: there are no characteristic lesions observed in organophosphate-insecticide poisoned animals. Pulmonary changes may be observed, including an increased bronchial secretions and pulmonary oedema. Pancreatitis may be present.

Treatment

If the ingestion has occurred within 2 hours, vomiting may be induced or gastric lavage performed, and then adsorbents administered.

Emetics:

(a)	Apomorphine	Dose:	0.05 mg/kg body weight i.v. or i.m.; 0.1 mg/kg body weight s.c.
(b)	Xylazine	Dose:	0.2 mg/kg body weight i.v.; 0.5–1 mg/kg body weight i.m. or s.c.
(c)	Ipecacuanha	Dose:	1–2 ml/kg body weight (maximum 20 ml) orally
(d)	Soda crystal.		

Adsorbents:

(a)	Activated charcoal	Dose:	2 g/kg body weight orally
(b)	BCK granules®	Dose:	6–18 g orally two or three times daily.

If there is a risk of dermal exposure, the animal should be thoroughly washed with a mild shampoo or detergent.

Further management is largely symptomatic; in particular, body temperature should be maintained and blood gases and electrolytes monitored and corrected. Rehydration may be required.

If sedation is required then diazepam may be given. Dose: 0.5 mg/kg body weight i.v. repeated every 10 minutes up to three times if needed.

Atropine should be given to reverse cholinergic effects. Dose: 0.2–2 mg/kg body weight (one-quarter of the dose given i.v. and the remainder s.c. or i.m.) repeated as required (usually every 45–90 minutes initially). Large doses may be required for effect.

Atropine has no effect on nicotinic receptors and will not counteract skeletal muscle tremors, weakness or neuromuscular paralysis.

Pralidoxime may be given in severe cases, preferably within the first 24 hours. Dose: 20 mg/kg i.m. or by slow i.v. injection (at a rate not exceeding 500 mg/

minute) two or three times daily. Pralidoxime is given as an adjunct to atropine therapy. Recovery with pralidoxime will be not be immediate (as with atropine) but gradual, over a period of 24–48 hours. In cases where initiation of therapy with pralidoxime is delayed, it should be started and continued until the animal is asymptomatic or unless no improvement in nicotinic signs (e.g. decrease in muscle tremors, weakness or paralysis) is seen after 24–36 hours of pralidoxime therapy.

Contra-indicated drugs

Phenothiazine sedatives and succinylcholine should be avoided because of the neuromuscular blocking activity, since they will exacerbate the toxicity of organophosphate insecticides. Antibiotics such as aminoglycosides (e.g. strepto-mycin, gentamicin, neomycin, kanamycin), polypeptides (e.g. polymixin A and B) and clindamycin should also be avoided, since they may have neuromuscular blocking effects. Benzodiazepines, opioids and barbiturates should be used cautiously because of their CNS depressant effects.

Laboratory investigations

Cholinesterase activity determination may be considered. It is advised that whole blood from unaffected animals should also be submitted as a control. Although not a uniformly reliable indicator, a decrease of 50% or more of normal activity generally indicates significant inhibition and in many cases the cholinesterase activity is less than 25% of normal.

Delayed effects

Treatment of delayed neurotoxicity is symptomatic and supportive. The effects are generally refractory to antidotal therapy.

References and further reading

VPIS (London) past cases up to 98/16754.

Bodgett D *et al.* (1996). How do I treat? Organophosphate toxicity. *Progress in Veterinary Neurology* **7(2)**, 56–57.

Fikes JD (1990). Organophosphate and carbamate insecticides. *Veterinary Clinics of North America: Small Animal Practice* **20(2)**, 353–367.

Maksimovic PN *et al.* (1991). Treatment of acute dichlorvos poisoning in dogs. *Acta Veterinaria Scandinavica*, Suppl. **87**, 347–348.

Mayer S (1990). Organophosphates. *In Practice* **12(6)**, 250–251.

Talcott PA and Dorman DC (1997). Pesticide exposures in companion animals. *Veterinary Medicine* **92(2)**, 167–181.

Paracetamol

Type of product

Paracetamol is an analgesic drug and is also a non-narcotic, with anti-pyretic properties similar to those of aspirin but without being anti-inflammatory. It has a good safety profile in humans when used at recommended dosages.

Presentation

Paracetamol is widely available in the UK as an 'over-the-counter' medication for human use. It is sold under many brand names in both tablet and liquid suspension preparations.

The dose of paracetamol in tablet preparations is variable but the most common strengths encountered are 120 mg and 500 mg. Liquid suspensions are also marketed under a variety of brand names and in varying strengths, though the most commonly encountered strengths are 120 mg/5 ml and 250 mg/5ml.

Many preparations on the market contain paracetamol in combination with other analgesic drugs, such as aspirin and opioids. Paracetamol may also be found in preparations containing antihistamines, decongestant drugs and caffeine.

Note: In the USA and Canada, paracetamol is called acetaminophen.

Occurrence of poisoning incidences

Since the launch of the VPIS in 1992, paracetamol has been among the most common drugs about which it has been consulted. Until 1996 some 1.9% of enquiries to the London centre involved paracetamol, with this percentage then rising to 2.5%. More than 80% of these enquiries usually involve canine cases, which predominantly occur as a result of accidental ingestion of packets left accessible to the animals.

Recommended dosage

In the UK, the drug is supplied for use in humans only.

There are **no** indications for use of this drug in veterinary medicine.

Toxicity

Dogs are susceptible to the effects of paracetamol. In particular, they are prone to development of liver damage and methaemoglobinaemia.

According to the literature:

- Dogs can tolerate 45 mg/kg body weight per day orally without development of clinical effects.
- Ingestion of 100 mg/kg produced no clinical effects.
- Oral doses of 200 mg/kg body weight may cause signs of toxicity to develop, including methaemoglobinaemia.
- A single oral dose of 500 mg/kg body weight has resulted in a methaemoglobinaemia greater than 50%.
- 500 mg/kg body weight has resulted in fatality.
- 1 g/kg body weight over 24 hours produced delayed hepatic failure (36 hours onset).

In the experience of the VPISLn:

- Doses of 330 mg/kg body weight and 555 mg/kg body weight have been ingested by dogs with no apparent clinical effects. In these cases, emesis was induced promptly and antidotal therapy given (VPISLn cases 85/33780 and 93/112924).
- A dog was presented 12 hours after ingestion of 545 mg/kg body weight of paracetamol with vomiting, diarrhoea and facial oedema. At 48 hours icterus and brown urine were noted. Acetylcysteine was given and the animal made a gradual but complete recovery (VPISLn case 93/26239).
- Doses of 285 mg/kg body weight and 330 mg/kg body weight have been associated with fatality. In both these cases the dogs were presented late. The first had haemorrhagic diarrhoea, dehydration and collapse and died despite supportive care and N-acetylcysteine administration (VPISLn case 95/22701). The other had vomiting, ataxia, tachycardia, tachypnoea, and haematuria. The animal required euthanasia (VPISLn case 95/72610).

Mechanism of toxicity

In all species, paracetamol is metabolised in the liver by glucuronidation, sulphation and oxidation. The glucuronide and sulphate conjugates are non-toxic and are excreted in bile and urine. In most species, the oxidation pathway is a very minor one and glucuronidation is the major pathway. This is true of the dog where glucuronidation metabolism occurs for 75% of an ingested dose. In dogs between 10 and 20% of an ingested dose will be metabolised by sulphation.

With increasing paracetamol dosing, both the sulphation and glucuronidation pathways become saturated as they are capacity limited processes. This results in more paracetamol being metabolised by oxidation.

At low paracetamol doses some 3–5% of the drug undergoes oxidation. This pathway, mediated by cytochrome P_{450}, involves N-hydroxylation, followed by spontaneous formation of N-acetyl-p-benzoquinoneimine, a highly reactive metabolite. Normally this is conjugated with reduced glutathione, then further metabolised to cysteine and mercaptopuric acid derivatives, which are non-toxic and which are excreted in urine. At low dosings this can be an effective and efficient detoxification pathway.

At higher paracetamol doses, when the glucuronidation and sulphation routes are saturated and paracetamol levels in blood and liver rise the oxidation pathway increases in activity. This results in increased production of N-acetyl-p-benzoquinoneimine, causing glutathione depletion in the liver and subsequently in red blood cells as the detoxification pathway is used. As glutathione becomes depleted the reactive N-acetyl-p-benzoquinoneimine binds covalently with amino acid residues of cellular macromolecules and proteins with subsequent cellular necrosis.

At higher doses paracetamol also inhibits glutathione synthesis, further restricting the capacity of this pathway to produce non-toxic metabolites.

Alternative metabolic pathways also allow accumulation of oxidising metabolites that may induce methaemoglobin formation, Heinz body formation and denaturation of erythrocyte membranes. Heinz bodies are denatured chains of haemoglobin with oxidised sulphydryl groups. They precipitate and migrate towards cell membranes where, perhaps due to alteration of membrane phospholipids, they render cells fragile. Haemolysis and restricted passage of erythrocytes through the microcirculation and spleen may result. Canine haemoglobin has four sulphydryl groups per molecule and is therefore susceptible to denaturation. Methaemoglobinaemia reduces oxygen carrying capacity. It is unclear whether methaemoglobinaemia is directly related to Heinz body formation.

In the presence of glutathione, methaemoglobin will be reduced to haemoglobin. However, when paracetamol levels are high, glutathione will be depleted and its synthesis reduced and hence insufficient quantities will be available for this reduction. Methaemoglobin accumulation occurs and, as it cannot bind oxygen, tissue hypoxia will result. Methaemoglobinaemia further pushes the oxidation dissociation curve to the left, impairing unloading of oxygen further exacerbating the anoxia. Methaemoglobinaemia normally only occurs when oxidative stress overwhelms erythrocyte capacity.

Hence glutathione availability is crucial in prevention of methaemoglobin and Heinz body formation. It can be seen that increased metabolism of paracetamol via the oxidative pathway is causative of the clinical picture following paracetamol administration. The characteristic picture in dogs is one of methaemoglobinaemia, cyanosis, anaemia and jaundice. Death usually occurs from progressive methaemoglobinaemia or from severe hepatic necrosis.

Kinetics and metabolism

Paracetamol is rapidly absorbed from the gastrointestinal tract under normal conditions. Clinical effects are normally apparent within 4 hours.

The various metabolic pathways are discussed in the above section on mechanism of toxicity. As the elimination pathways are capacity limited, the plasma half-life is dependent on dose. Experimentally determined half-lives have been recorded at 1.2 hours after paracetamol doses of 200 mg/kg body weight and 3.5 hours after 500 mg/kg body weight.

A paracetamol dosing of 200 mg/kg body weight in dogs produced a methaemoglobinaemia of 18.8% in 4 hours; 500 mg/kg body weight produced a 51.9% level.

Clinical effects

Clinical effects usually occur within 4–12 hours.

Early effects

Within 1–4 hours there may be progressive cyanosis, tachycardia, tachypnoea and dyspnoea, all of which are dependent on the degree of methaemoglobinaemia. Depression, vomiting, diarrhoea, anorexia, facial and paw oedema, pale mucous membranes, pruritus and hypothermia may also be evident. Haematuria, anaemia, and evidence of haemolysis may be present.

Less common effects include initial hyperactivity, depression, sedation, salivation, lacrimation, abdominal tenderness, ataxia and collapse.

Later effects

From 2–7 days there may be haemoglobinuria, intravascular haemolysis, icterus and other evidence of liver damage (e.g. raised alanine amino-transferase and bilirubin). Coma, convulsions and pulmonary oedema are sometimes reported and are poor prognostic signs.

Death from hepatic failure usually occurs between 2 and 6 days post-ingestion.

Laboratory diagnosis

There may be raised alanine aminotransferase, aspartate transaminase, alkaline phosphatase, total and direct bilirubin, and elevation of other liver enzymes indicative of icterus. Decreased packed cell volume, methaemo-globinaemia (chocolate blood colour of blood samples) and Heinz body formation may be evident. Haemoglobinuria, proteinuria, and bilirubinuria (dark brown urine colour) have all been reported. A metabolic acidosis with respiratory compensation has been reported.

Note: Biochemical abnormalities may take up to 2 weeks to return to normal.

Post-mortem findings

Hepatic centrilobular congestion and necrosis is characteristic in dogs. Peripheral degenerative changes in the liver include pericholangitis, mononuclear cell infiltrates, bile duct proliferation, biliary stasis and presence of vacuolated hepatocytes.

Pulmonary congestion and oedema are sometimes noted. Haemorrhagic congestion, oedema and petechiae renal cortex and medulla have been reported.

Unclotted plum/chocolate coloured blood, indicative of methaemoglobinaemia, will be present.

Treatment

Cases that present late are more at risk from the serious adverse/toxic effects.

Treatment is recommended if more than 150 mg/kg body weight has been exceeded.

If within 2 hours of ingestion induce, vomiting or perform gastric lavage, and then administer adsorbents.

Emetics:

(a)	Apomorphine	Dose:	0.05 mg/kg body weight i.v. or i.m.; 0.1 mg/kg body weight s.c.
(b)	Xylazine	Dose:	0.2 mg/kg body weight i.v.; 0.5–1 mg/kg body weight i.m. or s.c.
(c)	Ipecacuanha	Dose:	1–2 ml/kg body weight (maximum 20 ml) orally
(d)	Soda crystal.		

Adsorbents:

(a)	Activated charcoal	Dose:	2 g/kg body weight orally
(b)	BCK granules®	Dose:	6–18 g orally.

Note

Adsorbents should not be given where antidotes are to be administered orally because it may reduce their efficacy.

If the animal is cyanosed then oxygen should be administered. In addition, there are several antidotal therapies that may be employed.

Antidotal therapy

Probably the most widely used antidote in paracetamol poisoning is N-acetylcysteine because it can significantly reduce the toxicity of the drug by a variety of mechanisms. First, it is a precursor of glutathione. On administration it is hydrolysed to form L-cysteine, which provides substrate for glutathione synthesis in red blood cells and the liver. Glutathione cannot be given directly, as it is not readily taken up by cells. Second, it acts directly on the reactive metabolite resulting from the cytochrome P_{450}-mediated oxidation of paracetamol, N-acetyl-p-benzoquinoneimine, to form an acetylcysteine conjugate that can be excreted, although this reaction is slow. Third, it is oxidised in the liver to form sulphate, thereby increasing the capacity of the sulphation pathway.

Methionine is a precursor for glutathione and sulphate and has some use. It may be given where N-acetylcysteine is unavailable or used in conjunction with N-acetylcysteine therapy.

Ascorbic acid can be given to reduce methaemoglobin to haemoglobin as it is a good non-enzymatic reductant, although the reaction does occur slowly. There is some evidence to suggest it may also scavenge N-acetyl-p-benzoquinoneimine before it binds to proteins, possibly reducing it back to paracetamol. This certainly happens *in vitro*, though there is debate as to whether it happens *in vivo*. It may be given in combination with the other antidotes.

Administration of sodium sulphate increases sulphate for conjugation, thereby increasing capacity of the sulphation route of metabolism. It may be used in combination with the other antidotes.

In cases of severe methaemoglobinaemia, methylene blue may be used. This drug increases reduction of methaemoglobin. It is reduced to leucomethylene blue by an NADPH-dependent methaemoglobin reductase. The leucomethylene blue then reduces the oxidised haem iron to its normal state. However, it should be used with caution as high doses can themselves cause methaemoglobinaemia or haemolytic anaemia.

Regimens for antidotes:

(a) N-acetylcysteine   Dose: Either 140 mg/kg body weight orally, wait 6 hours, then 70 mg/kg body weight orally every 6–8 hours for 36 hours or more, dependent on the clinical condition of the animal (some sources state it can be given for up to 72 hours) or 280 mg/kg body weight by slow i.v. injection over 6 hours, then 70 mg/kg body weight orally every 6–8 hours for 36 hours or more dependent on the clinical condition of the animal (some sources state it can be given for up to 72 hours).

Note

The second method should be employed if adsorbents have previously been given.

(b) Methionine   Dose: 70 mg/kg body weight orally every 6–8 hours, up to 24 hours.

Note

If adsorbents have previously been given, a 6-hour period should elapse before administration is started.

(c) Ascorbic acid	Dose:	30 mg/kg body weight i.v. every 6–8 hours until no cyanosis is present.
(d) Sodium sulphate	Dose:	1.6% solution; 50 mg/kg body weight i.v. every 4 hours, up to 24 hours.
(e) Methylene blue	Dose:	1–5 mg/kg body weight by slow intravenous injection.

Other care

Management is otherwise symptomatic and supportive, with particular care being taken to ensure adequate hydration and maintenance of body temperature. Use of heat pads or other warming methods have been required in some cases.

Urea, electrolytes and blood gases should be checked if possible and corrected where necessary. The animal should also be monitored for evidence of liver damage, anaemia and haemolysis. If there is evidence of severe haemolysis, significant decrease in packed cell volume, or severe anaemia then whole blood transfusions may be required.

It is recommended that blood counts are monitored for at least 1 week post-therapy.

References and further reading

VPIS (London) past cases up to 97/65219.

Harvey JW *et al.* (1986). Hematologic abnormalities associated with chronic acetaminophen administration in a dog. *Journal of the American Veterinary Medical Association* **189(10)**, 1334–1335.

Hjelle JJ and Grauer GF (1986). Acetaminophen-induced toxicosis in dogs and cats. *Journal of the American Veterinary Medical Association* **188(7)**, 742–746.

Kolf-Clauw M and Keck G (1994). Paracetamol poisoning in dogs and cats. *European Journal of Companion Animal Practice* **4**, 85–92.

Kore AM (1997). Over-the-counter analgesic drug toxicoses in small animals. *Veterinary Medicine* **92(2)**, 158–165.

Marcella KL (1983). Acetaminophen poisoning in cats and man. *Journal of the American Veterinary Medical Association* **183(8)**, 836.

Mayer S (1991). Poison – paracetamol. *In Practice* **13(1)**, 37.

Ortega L *et al.* (1985). Acetaminophen-induced fulminant hepatic failure in dogs. *Hepatology* **5(4)**, 673–676.

Savides MC *et al.* (1984). The toxicity and biotransformation of single doses of acetaminophen in dogs and cats. *Toxicology and Applied Pharmacology* **74**, 26–34.

Schlesinger DP (1995). Methaemoglobinaemia and anemia in a dog with acetaminophen toxicity. *Canadian Veterinary Journal* **36**, 515–517.

Thursby-Pelham C (1996). Peculiar drug poisonings in pets. *In Practice* **18(10)**, 478–487.

Villar D, Buck WB and Gonzalez JM (1998). Ibuprofen, aspirin and acetaminophen toxicosis and treatment in dogs and cats. *Veterinary and Human Toxicology* **40(3)**, 156–161.

Paraquat

Type of product

Paraquat is a non-selective, foliage-applied contact herbicide first marketed in 1962. Since 1972, the UK Poisons Act has restricted the purchase of concentrates containing >5% paraquat to farmers and horticulturalists only.

Presentation

Paraquat is available as an aqueous concentrate and also in granular formulations; all require dilution with or dissolving in water before use. Products for agricultural use are generally supplied in a liquid form (typically 20% paraquat), although there are a few granular formulations available. In the UK, paraquat is readily available for domestic use in a granular form, which is made up with water for use. These domestic formulations are <5% w/w paraquat ion, generally 2.5% w/w. The manufacturers recommend that the maximum strength used in application should not exceed 0.5% (5 g/L). Some products may also contain other herbicides.

A stenching agent (1975) and an emetic (1977) were added to liquid paraquat products to reduce the risk of accidental poisoning. The emetic (a potent centrally-acting triazolo-pyrimidine code-named PP796) is in a concentration that would cause vomiting if the minimum potential lethal dose of paraquat formulation for humans had been ingested.

Occurrence of poisoning incidences

The VPIS London centre receives many enquiries concerning paraquat each year, representing approximately 1.2% of the annual enquiry number. These enquiries predominantly involve exposures in dogs, which are most frequently due to malicious poisonings of animals by neighbours. Paraquat is one of the agents that most frequently results in fatalities in the experience of the VPIS. Each year between 10 and 20% of the cases involving paraquat referred have a fatal outcome.

Not all cases result from intentional poisoning. Some occur from ingestion of recently treated plant material or of the neat preparations by animals. In plant, paraquat acts by alteration of enzyme systems and disruption of photosynthesis. After application the plant begins to dry and the leaves drop within 1–7 days. The portion absorbed by plants is retained until the leaves drop and this presents a hazard to animals eating large quantities of recently sprayed vegetation. Paraquat is rapidly inactivated by and strongly binds to soil.

Toxicity

The classic picture of paraquat poisoning in dogs is vomiting following by progressive respiratory distress. In many cases, the source and timing of paraquat exposure is not known and paraquat is assumed to be the agent responsible for illness. Recovery from poisoning is rare and prognosis is poor, especially if there is onset of severe dyspnoea prognosis is poor.

According to the literature:

- There are reports of poisoning in dogs who have eaten carcasses baited with paraquat to kill foxes. In one reported case a dog ate the vomit of another dog, which had been observed leaving a carcass of a calf baited with paraquat. Both dogs developed dyspnoea and were put down.
- The LD_{50} in dogs is 25–50 mg/kg body weight.
- A concentration of 36 ppm in food caused no ill effects in dogs. A dose of 85 ppm in food over 27 months or 170 ppm for 2 months resulted in respiratory failure and death.
- The expected concentration in grass from the recommended application rate is 75–150 ppm.

In the experience of the VPISLn:

- About 25% of cases reported to VPISLn are cases of malicious poisoning and about 40% are due to ingestion of recently treated vegetation.
- Over 70% of cases involving products for professional use result in fatality.

Mechanism of toxicity

Paraquat was originally used as a redox indicator (known as methyl viologen) and it is this ability to continually undergo redox cycling that accounts for its toxicity. The exact mechanisms of toxicity are not fully understood, but are thought to be a combination of NADPH depletion and free radical formation. Paraquat undergoes a NADPH-dependent reduction to form the free radical. This free radical reacts with molecular oxygen to reform the cation and produce a superoxide free radical and will do so continually in the presence of NADPH and oxygen. The superoxide free radicals then disrupt cell function and structure, damaging them by lipid peroxidation, which may cause cell death. Cellular NADPH becomes depleted, partly from continual redox cycling of paraquat and also from its requirement in detoxification of lipid hydroperoxides and of hydrogen peroxide, which is formed in the presence of superoxide dismutase.

In massive overdose paraquat can cause death within hours of ingestion from multi-organ failure. Lower doses can cause lung damage, which may result in death days or weeks later. The lung is the main target for paraquat toxicity due to active, energy-dependent uptake by alveolar type I and II cells; paraquat seems to produce an acute damaging phase in the lung followed by a reparative phase in which extensive fibrosis occurs.

Kinetics and metabolism

Paraquat is rapidly but poorly absorbed from the gastrointestinal tract and concentrates in the lungs. Metabolism is minimal (except for the redox reactions described above) and is primarily excreted unchanged in the urine. Paraquat may be detected in urine for up to 2 days after ingestion and sometimes for up to 7 days.

Clinical effects

Onset and duration: vomiting and depression start after 1–3 days, respiratory signs after 2–7 days. Death may occur within 8 days. If the animal survives for more than 7 days post-exposure there may be partial recovery over days 7–10 with progressive respiratory distress, which may continue until death 10–21 days post-exposure. Recovery in animals that survive may be prolonged (7 weeks of intensive care in one case).

Note: Systemic toxicity may occur following dermal exposure, particularly with the concentrated formulations.

The initial clinical effects include vomiting, diarrhoea, salivation, haematemesis, abdominal tenderness, lethargy, anorexia, inappetence, ulceration of mouth and tongue, dullness, ataxia, pyrexia, polydipsia and dehydration.

In severe cases, the animals may develop tachypnoea, sometimes with mild bradycardia. This progresses to severe dyspnoea, which is usually the most dominant feature and may be accompanied by tachycardia and cyanosis. On radiography of the chest, there is usually a variety of infiltrative changes, which are often mild compared with the degree of respiratory distress. Pneumomediastinum occurs in about 25% of cases. Convulsions and renal failure may also occur.

Biochemistry values may indicate dehydration, a neutrophilic and monocytic leucocytosis, uraemia and hypokalaemia.

Post-mortem findings

There may be dark congested and haemorrhagic lungs with bronchioles and alveoli dilated with bilious emphysematous areas. Commonly, there is necrosis of bronchioles and alveolar epithelium with the greatest effects noticeable in type I pneumocytes.

Other findings include renal tubular necrosis, focal myocardial necrosis, adrenal necrosis, and duodenal congestion. The spleen may be enlarged.

Treatment

Emptying the stomach is not worthwhile due to rapid absorption. Adsorbents should be given as soon as possible, though these are probably only of benefit up to 6 hours post-ingestion.

Adsorbents:

(a) Activated charcoal   Dose: 2 g/kg body weight orally

(b) BCK granules®   Dose: 6–18 g orally two or three times daily.

It is essential to thoroughly wash any animal that may have had paraquat on the skin using soap and water.

Anti-emetics may be required.

(a) Metoclopramide   Dose: 0.5–1 mg/kg body weight orally, s.c. or i.m. every 6–8 hours; 1–2 mg/kg body weight per day by slow i.v. infusion

(b) Acepromazine   Dose: 0.03–0.1 mg/kg body weight i.v., i.m., or s.c. (use lower dose if giving i.v.); 1–3 mg/kg body weight orally.

Diazepam may be given if there is any convulsant activity (dose: 0.5 mg/kg body weight i.v. repeated every 10 minutes up to three times if needed).

Care should also be taken to maintain fluid balance and monitor renal and respiratory function. It has been suggested that administration of oxygen should be avoided but the avidity of paraquat for oxygen is such that it is very unlikely to make any difference. There is no specific antidote. Numerous regimens of various drugs have been tried in human cases of paraquat poisoning and all have failed to alter the outcome. Treatment is symptomatic and supportive.

Investigative

The paraquat urine spot test may be useful in the early stages of a poisoning to confirm exposure. It is also possible to measure paraquat concentrations in blood.

Urine spot test: Add 100 mg sodium dithionite to 10 ml of 1M sodium hydroxide solution. Add 1 ml of this to 1 ml of urine. A blue–green colour indicates a positive result. It is usually only positive within the first 48 hours after exposure (depending on the amount ingested) but has been detected up to 7 days later in some cases.

References and further reading

VPIS (London) past cases up to 97/76203.

Barton M and Gaskell CJ (1982). Poisoning after illegal use of paraquat bait. *Veterinary Record* **110**, 565.

Darke PGG *et al.* (1977). Acute respiratory distress in the dog associated with paraquat poisoning. *Veterinary Record* **100**, 275–277.

Darke P (1992). Paraquat. *In Practice* **14(2)**, 66.

Hampson ECGM *et al.* (1990). Efficacy of single or repeated hemoperfusion in a canine model of paraquat poisoning. *Journal of Pharmacology and Experimental Therapeutics* **254(2)**, 732–740.

Longstaffe JA *et al.* (1981). Paraquat poisoning in dogs and cats – differences between accidental and malicious poisoning. *Journal of Small Animal Practice* **22**, 153–156.

O'Sullivan SP (1989). Paraquat poisoning in the dog. *Journal of Small Animal Practice* **30**, 361–364.

Quick MP *et al.* (1990). Acute and sub-acute paraquat poisoning in a pack of foxhounds. *Journal of the Forensic Science Society* **30(6)**, 37–376.

Phenolphthalein

Type of product

Phenolphthalein is a laxative drug.

Presentation

Many preparations are available for human use. Some contain phenolphthalein in combination with sennosides and bisacodyl. Tablets are of varying strengths. Some contain up to 130 mg phenolphthalein. Some preparations are presented as 'chocolate' tablets. This is flavouring only.

Occurrence of poisoning incidences

Since 1992, the VPIS London centre has received up to 10 enquiries per year about accidental ingestions of phenolphthalein by dogs. Despite ingestion of substantial quantities in some cases, all remained asymptomatic, except one dog, who was described as lethargic.

Recommended dosage

Phenolphthalein is not recommended for use in dogs.

Toxicity

No fatal case data in dogs has been reported. Laxative effect reportedly only occurs in primates, pigs and some birds.

Clinical effects

None are anticipated.

Treatment

No treatment is necessary, even for very substantial ingestions. Note: Some preparations are presented as 'chocolate tablets'. This is a flavouring only, and therefore there is no risk of effects from theobromine alkaloids.

Reference

VPIS (London) past cases up to 98/32076.

Phenoxy acid herbicides

Type of product

Phenoxy derivative herbicides are selective to broad-leaved plants, and thus are often used as lawn weed killers.

Substances include:

2,4-D	(2,4-dichlorophenoxyacetic acid)
2,4,5-T	(2,4,5-trichlorophenoxyacetic acid)
2,4-DB	(4(2,4-dichlorophenoxy) butyric acid)
MCPA	(4-chloro-o-tolyloxy acetic acid)
MCPB	(2-(2-methyl-4-chlorophenoxy) butyric acid)
MCPP	(mecoprop; 2,2-chloro-o-tolyloxy propionic acid)
Dicamba	
Dichlorprop.	

Presentation

There are a number of products that contain phenoxy acid herbicides. Some are presented as 'feed and weed' preparations. Products may be in granular or liquid form. These chemicals are not very soluble in water and solvents may be present in liquid formulations.

Occurrence of poisoning incidences

Since the launch of the VPIS in 1992, the London centre has received 45–60 enquiries about phenoxy acid herbicides each year. Enquiries about these pesticides represent about 2.5% of the total cases reported each year. Most of these enquiries involve dogs and the herbicides most frequently implicated in these cases are 2,4-D, mecoprop and dicamba.

Toxicity

These compounds do not differ greatly in their toxicity; the LD_{50} for most species is in the range 100–500 mg/kg body weight. However, dogs appear to be more sensitive to phenoxy acid herbicides than other mammals.

According to the literature:

- The LD_{50} of 2,4-D in dogs is 100 mg/kg body weight.
- Multiple doses of 20 mg/kg of 2,4-D for approximately 3 weeks or 25 mg/kg for 6 days were lethal in dogs.
- 250 ppm of dicamba fed to dogs caused mild hepatic jaundice and no other adverse health effects.

- 2560 ppm of MCPA or MCPP acutely fed to dogs caused anaemia and decreased weight gains.
- 640 ppm of MCPA or MCPP chronically fed to dogs caused decreased weight gains.

In the experience of VPISLn:

Several fatal cases have been reported. In one case, the dog ingested grass sprayed with 2,4-D, dicamba and ioxynil. The dog became unwell over 3 days with tachycardia, bradypnoea, haematemesis, bloody diarrhoea and depression. The dog improved initially but died 18 hours after admission (VPISLn case 91/26244). In a second case, the dog ate 2,4-D, mecoprop and bromadiolone (an anticoagulant rodenticide). The clinical effects developed over 1–2 weeks and were ataxia, weakness, jaundice, anaemia and pyrexia (VPISLn case 93/50139). Another dog of 10 kg body weight died 5 days after ingestion of 2,4-D. Clinical effects included collapse and convulsions (VPISLn case 95/153208).

Mechanism of toxicity

The mode of action of poisoning of phenoxy acid herbicides is not understood. The gastric effects are probably due to their acidity. They may uncouple oxidative phosphorylation. This results in the energy that would be stored as ATP being dissipated as heat. In dogs, phenoxy acid derivatives may also directly affect muscle membranes. They are also known to depress ribonuclease synthesis and to increase the number of hepatic peroxisomes, but the significance of these effects to the toxicity of these compounds is unknown. In plants these compounds act as hormones; they have no hormonal action in animals.

Kinetics and metabolism

Phenoxy acid derivatives are readily absorbed from the gastrointestinal tract. They are protein-bound and rapidly distributed to the liver, kidneys and brain. There is some metabolism of these compounds; esters are metabolised by hydrolysis and small amounts may be conjungated to glycine or taurine. The majority is excreted unchanged in the urine and dogs excrete phenoxy acid derivates relatively slowly. Excretion is enhanced if the urine is alkaline, because these compounds are acidic.

Clinical effects

Commonly observed effects include inappetence, anorexia, ataxia, salivation, vomiting, haematemesis, abdominal pain and diarrhoea, which may be bloody. Animals may be polydipsic. Lethargy, depression, myotonia, and weakness, particularly of hind legs, have also been reported. Some dogs have collapsed. Animals may be bradycardic or tachycardic, and have respiratory distress or depression.

In severe cases, opisthotonus, coma and convulsions may occur.

Laboratory analysis may show changes in alkaline phosphatase, lactate dehydrogenase and creatinine kinase concentrations consistent with liver, kidney and muscle damage.

Post-mortem findings

Post-mortem studies have revealed necrotic lesions and ulcers of the oral mucosa, signs of irritation of the gastrointestinal tract and sometimes of the small intestine, liver necrosis and degeneration of renal tubules

Treatment

Emesis is best avoided because of the risk of aspiration of the volatile solvents present in some preparations.

Adsorbents may be given.

(a) Activated charcoal	Dose:	2 g/kg body weight orally
(b) BCK granules®	Dose:	6–18 g orally two or three times daily.

Any animal with dermal exposure should be thoroughly washed with detergent (these compounds are poorly soluble in water).

Treatment is symptomatic and supportive as there is no specific antidote. Avoid oil or paraffin cathartics as these may enhance absorption. Ensure adequate hydration. Anti-emetics such as metoclopramide or acepromazine may be given if necessary.

Anti-emetics

(a) Metoclopramide	Dose:	0.5–1 mg/kg body weight orally, s.c. or i.m. every 6–8 hours; 1–2 mg/kg body weight per day by slow i.v. infusion
(b) Acepromazine	Dose:	0.03–0.1 mg/kg body weight i.v., i.m., or s.c. (use lower dose if giving i.v.); 1–3 mg/kg body weight orally.

Diazepam may be given if there is any convulsant activity. Dose: 0.5 mg/kg body weight i.v. repeated every 10 minutes up to three times if needed.

Blood transfusions may be necessary in animals with severe anaemia.

References and further reading

VPIS (London) cases up to 97/167334.

Cooper BS (1987). Animal toxicoses associated with herbicides and fertilisers. In *Veterinary Clinical Toxicology, Proceedings No. 103*, Post-graduate Committee in Veterinary Science, University of Sydney, pp. 189–203.

Plastic explosive compounds

Type of product

Various different chemical compounds are used as plastic explosives.

Examples include:

- Semtex
- RDX (Royal Defence Explosive – major ingredient cyclonite)
- Cyclonite (cyclotrimethylenetrinitramine) – a compound widely used in warfare since World War II.
- Composition PE-4 (major ingredients cyclonite, paraffin and a bonding agent)
- Composition C-4 (major ingredient is cyclonite 91%, mixed with polyisobutylene 2.1%, motor oil 1.6%, and di-(2-ethyl-hexyl) sebacate 5.3%) – this was the explosive most commonly used in the Vietnam conflict.

Presentation

Their general characteristics are that they are malleable solids, usually burn under normal conditions without exploding, and are relatively insensitive to friction or impact and are therefore easily transported without undue precaution being merited.

They require a blasting cap to detonate.

Cyclonite is described as being a colourless crystal that is very insoluble in water and most body fluids.

Occurrence of poisoning incidences

Since the launch of the VPIS in 1992, a few enquiries have been received about ingestion of plastic explosive compounds by dogs. The animals that have been exposed to these agents are usually being trained for military or police purposes and have accidentally ingested them during routine training. No cases reported to the VPIS have resulted in fatality, although the clinical effects have been classified as serious or severe. VPIS cases have involved PE-4, C-4 and Semtex.

Toxicity

According to the literature:

- In an experimental case involving PE-4 in a 27-month-old, 26 kg, cross-bred female dog an oral dose of 3.85 mg/kg body weight caused no apparent effects within 2.5 hours. A further dose was given, bringing the total dose to 33.85 mg/kg body weight, with eventual fatality. The authors estimated an effective fatal dosing of 14 mg/kg body weight (see case report below).

In the experience of VPISLn

- A Retriever ingested C-4 on a training exercise. The animal quickly developed lethargy, ataxia, trembling, and fitting and also haematuria. After supportive management, including diazepam administration, the animal recovered in 48 hours (VPISLn case 91/48600).
- An English Springer ate an unknown quantity of PE-4. Within 1 hour the animal was confused, hyperaesthesic, vomiting and fitting. With diazepam and supportive care the animal recovered (VPISLn case 91/90365).

Kinetics and metabolism

Absorption would appear to be rapid, as clinical effects usually occur within 2 hours. However, cyclonite is reportedly insoluble in most body fluids.

Case report

Following a case involving PE-4 in a dog where the animal survived, De Cramer and Short (1992) experimentally poisoned a 27-month-old, 26 kg, cross-bred bitch with 100 mg of PE-4 (a dose of 3.85 mg/kg body weight) with no effect within 2.5 hours. They then administered another 780 mg (total dose 33.85 mg/kg body weight). After 5 hours (7.5 hours after initial dosing) the animal developed severe congestion of mucous membranes, pyrexia, tachycardia, hyperventilation, hyperaesthesia, light tremors and then epileptiform convulsions. At 8 hours after the initial dosing the animal displayed generalised seizures lasting 3–5 minutes, separated by periods of about 10–25 minutes where the animal would gradually become more hypersensitive and congested before fitting and then remaining calm for a short while before the 'cycle' started again. These periods became progressively shorter until at 15–18 hours post-initial ingestion the animal became semi-comatose, then comatose, dyspnoeic and finally died.

Post-mortem revealed generalised congestion, hepatomegaly, pulmonary oedema, numerous petechial haemorrhages in the pancreas, severe congestion of both liver and kidneys and hydropic degeneration of the kidneys. Of the 880 mg administered 512 mg was found in the stomach content. Assuming non-selective absorption of cyclonite from the PE-4 mixture, the authors calculated an effective dosing of approximately 14 mg/kg of PE-4 resulted in fatality – an amount described by the authors as 'the volume of two peas'. Since little data are available on the absorption kinetics and bioavailability of cyclonite from PE-4, this experiment indicates a fatal dosing in the range 14–34 mg/kg body weight.

Clinical effects

They may have a very rapid onset – in one case involving cyclonite a dog developed fitting, vomiting, hyperaesthesia and apparent confusion within 1 hour of ingestion.

Clinical effects commonly reported include ataxia and lethargy in the initial stages, excessive salivation and respiratory distress, congestion of mucous membranes, vomiting, hyperventilation, excitability, tremors, hyperaesthesia, and severe and prolonged epileptiform convulsions that may have a duration of 6 hours or more. Fits may have a duration of 3 minutes or more and may be separated by periods of 10–30 minutes during which the animal may be initially calm and then gradually become more hyperaesthesic and tremorous until fitting recommences. Untreated cases may continue to fit until 18 hours post-ingestion.

Haematuria has been reported in one VPISLn case (91/48600).

Ingestion might also cause urinary incontinence, hepatic and renal impairment characterised by oliguria, haematuria, proteinuria, increased blood urea nitrogen, raised aminotransferase and serum bilirubin levels.

Post-mortem findings

Generalised congestion, hepatomegaly, pulmonary oedema, numerous petechial haemorrhages in the pancreas, severe congestion of both liver and kidneys and hydropic degeneration of the kidneys can be displayed at post-mortem.

Treatment

Dogs should be observed for a minimum of 4 hours following ingestion of any quantity.

The use of emetics is contra-indicated owing to the potential for fitting to occur.

If the animals develop clinical effects then it is advisable to anaesthetise or sedate the dog to control the convulsant activity (see later) and to allow a gastric lavage to be performed if considered appropriate, although this is probably only worthwhile within 2 hours of ingestion. Adsorbents may be administered at this stage also.

Adsorbents:

(a) Activated charcoal   Dose: 2 g/kg body weight orally
(b) BCK granules®   Dose: 6–18 g orally two or three times daily.

If convulsions occur or the animal becomes markedly hyperaesthesic then there are two preferred ways of managing cases.

1. Keep the dogs sedated but still slightly hyperaesthesic and in control of their vital reflexes until the clinical effects are seen to resolve and then allow the

animal to slowly recover. Continued sedation may be necessary for over 6 hours in some cases.

2. Alternatively, cases that present with severe symptomatology could be placed under deep anaesthesia for 6–8 hours, then the dogs allowed to come round, with resumption of anaesthesia if clinical effects reappear as the animal recovers. During this time, body fluids need to be maintained by alternating lactated Ringers and dextrose saline drips.

Drugs best suited for these purposes are:

(a) Diazepam
(b) Pentobarbitone

Doses recommended:

(a) Diazepam	2–5 mg/kg body weight given by i.v. injection in 5–10 mg doses followed by 2–5 mg/hour in 5% glucose by slow i.v. infusion
(b) Pentobarbitone	25–30 mg/kg body weight by slow intravenous infusion.

Note: Acepromazine may also be considered, although it is thought to be less safe as it lowers the threshold for convulsions and seizure activity and is therefore not recommended for animals with a history of epileptiform seizures. Therefore, its use is best avoided in these cases.

To prevent development of pulmonary oedema it is advisable to turn the dog every couple of hours while under the anaesthetic/sedative.

Lactated Ringer's solution has been recommended for animals that are acidotic and/or dehydrated. Frusemide has been given to enhance renal clearance in some cases. Both vitamins and antibiotics have been given in past cases.

If the animal is salivating excessively then atropine may be given. Dose: 30–50 μg/kg body weight given s.c.

References and further reading

VPIS (London) past cases up to 98/10008.

Berry AP, Arbuckle JBR and Nicol J (1983). Cyclonite poisoning in a dog. *Veterinary Record* **113**, 449.

De Cramer KGM and Short RP (1992). Plastic explosive poisoning in dogs. *Journal of the South African Veterinary Association* **63(1)**, 30–31.

Croft PG (1983). Cyclonite poisoning in a dog. *Veterinary Record* **113**, 477.

Harrell-Bruder B and Hutchins KL (1995). Seizures caused by ingestion of composition C-4. *Annals of Emergency Medicine* **26**, 746–748.

Littlewood JD (1983). Cyclonite poisoning in a dog. *Veterinary Record* **113**, 503.

Stone MAJ et al. (1969). Toxic effects following ingestion of C-4 plastic explosive. *Archives of Internal Medicine* **124**, 726–730.

Pyracantha

The plant

The common name for Pyracantha is firethorn and the plant belongs to the Rosaceae family.

This common evergreen shrub grows up to 3 m high, and has thorny branches and small, oval-shaped, glossy dark-green leaves with serrated edges. The plant flowers from May to September with small clusters of white/cream flowers. The bright orange/red ovoid shaped fruits ripen from August to March and contain tiny brown seeds.

Occurrence of poisoning incidences

Since the launch of the VPIS, the centre in London has received a small number of enquiries each year regarding ingestion of Pyracantha. All these enquiries have involved dogs. A few dogs have displayed mild clinical effects but most have remained asymptomatic. One fatal case in an adult German Shepherd dog was attributed to ingestion of a large part of a Pyracantha bush. However, no post-mortem study was performed, and therefore Pyracantha poisoning could not be confirmed as the cause of death (VPISLn case 96/164507).

Toxicity

The plant is considered of low toxicity.

Mechanism of toxicity

Pyracantha contains cyanogenic glycosides. These are not present in high enough concentrations to cause more than mild gastrointestinal effects, even when very substantial quantities of the plant have been consumed.

Clinical effects

Clinical effects are rare. Ingestion of large numbers of berries or quantities of plant material might result in vomiting, diarrhoea, salivation and rarely abdominal tenderness.

Treatment

Gastric decontamination using gastric lavage, emesis or adsorbents is not necessary as the berries are of low toxicity and if a significant quantity are ingested vomiting usually occurs spontaneously. Use of metoclopramide may be considered if vomiting is severe. Metoclopramide dose: 0.5–1 mg/kg body weight orally, s.c. or i.m. every 6–8 hours; 1–2 mg/kg body weight per day by slow i.v. infusion.

Reference

VPIS (London) past cases up to 97/102544.

Pyrethrins and pyrethroids

Type of product

Pyrethrins (jasmolin I and II, cinerin I and II, pyrethrin I and II) are naturally occurring esters of chrysanthemic acid and pyrethric acid, which are extracted from the flowers of *Chrysanthemum cinerariaefolium*.

Pyrethroids (allethrin, alphacypermethrin, bioresmethrin, cypermethrin, deltamethrin, fenvalerate, permethrin, phenothrin, resmethrin, tetramethrin) are synthetic pyrethrins.

Pyrethrins and pyrethroids are used as insecticides for the treatment of ectoparasitic infestation. They are used in cats, dogs, sheep, cattle, poultry, horses, goats and humans.

Presentation

Pyrethroids and pyrethrins are used in dogs for the control of fleas and lice. Preparations are available as dusting powders, shampoos and sprays.

Note: Dogs may also be exposed to agrochemical preparations not designed for veterinary use; some of these may contain other constituents, including other insecticides and solvents. Piperonyl butoxide is often added to insecticidal preparations as a synergist (it delays the metabolism of the insecticide and increases the toxicity).

Occurrence of poisoning incidences

Since 1992, the London centre of the VPIS has received between 10 and 50 enquiries per annum regarding pyrethroids and pyrethrins in animals. Approximately 30% of these involve dogs. Intoxication either occurs as a result of ingestion of products or through over-zealous application of insecticide preparations to the coats of dogs. There appears to be a degree of individual susceptibility.

Toxicity may arise from self-grooming of treated hair. Occasionally, toxicity may arise from animals being in close association with or grooming treated animals.

Recommended dosage

This varies with the individual preparation.

Toxicity

In the experience of the VPISLn:

- A 9-week-old Collie cross was treated dermally with a powder insecticide containing pyrethrins and piperonyl butoxide. Within 5 hours the animal developed profuse salivation, dyspnoea and abdominal tenderness. The animal later developed acute respiratory distress and pulmonary oedema. Despite aggressive oxygen therapy and supportive care the animal died 13 hours post-exposure (VPISLn case 91/42116).
- A 2-month-old Yorkshire Terrier was treated with a powder insecticide containing permethrin. Within 2 hours the puppy was shaking, salivating, and then convulsing. The animal was hospitalised but later collapsed and died (VPISLn case 96/133486).

Mechanism of toxicity

The toxic effects of pyrethroids and pyrethrins are due to alteration of the kinetics of voltage-dependent sodium channels in nerve membranes, which causes repetitive discharges or membrane depolarisation. Some pyrethroids may also inhibit gamma aminobutyric acid (GABA) receptors. This inhibits the GABA$_A$-receptor mediated chloride ion influx, the physiological function of which is to induce pre-synaptic inhibition. Loss of this inhibition can lead to hyperexcitability of nervous tissue and may be the mechanism by which these compounds produce convulsions.

In mammals, pyrethrins and pyrethroids are rapidly biotransformed and detoxified by ester hydrolysis or oxidation. As a result, these compounds are of relatively low toxicity in mammals. Also, the activity of these compounds on sodium channels is negatively correlated to temperature and the greater toxicity in insects may also be an effect of the lower body temperature of insects.

Note: Non-specific plasma esterases are important for detoxification of most pyrethroids and pyrethrins (except allethrin and pyrethrum). Organophosphorous insecticides inhibit these enzymes and simultaneous exposure to these insecticides will increase the toxicity of pyrethrins and pyrethroids.

Clinical effects

Onset is usually within 1–3 hours, sometimes up to 12 hours. Effects may have a duration of 1–3 days.

Note: Simultaneous exposure to organophosphate insecticides may increase the toxicity of pyrethroids and pyrethrins (see above). Piperonyl butoxide, often added as a synergist to delay metabolism and increase toxicity in insects, produces effects similar to that of pyrethrins and pyrethrins.

Vomiting, diarrhoea, salivation, ataxia, tremor, incoordination, twitching, dilated pupils, tachycardia, hyperexcitability, hyperaesthesia, thirst, pyrexia, hyperpnoea, muscle weakness and fasciculation and convulsions have all been reported. Respiratory distress, probably due to weakness of respiratory muscles, may occur.

Some compounds cause paraesthesia, for example shaking of feet when they are dry.

Treatment

If within 2 hours of ingestion, induce vomiting or perform gastric lavage, and then administer adsorbents.

Emetics:

(a) Apomorphine   Dose: 0.05 mg/kg body weight i.v. or i.m.;
                                                    0.1 mg/kg body weight s.c.

(b) Xylazine   Dose: 0.2 mg/kg body weight i.v.;
                                                    0.5–1 mg/kg body weight i.m. or s.c.

(c) Ipecacuanha   Dose: 1–2 ml/kg body weight (maximum 20 ml) orally

(d) Soda crystal.

Adsorbents:

(a) Activated charcoal   Dose: 2 g/kg body weight orally
(b) BCK granules   Dose: 6–18 g orally two–three times daily.

Treatment thereafter is essentially symptomatic and supportive.

If the exposure is dermal, the dog should be washed with lukewarm water and detergent. The use of very warm water should be avoided as this increased dermal perfusion and may result in increase, dermal absorption. Copious amounts of detergent should be used because pyrethrins and pyrethroids are not soluble in water. Following washing, collaring is recommended to prevent further grooming.

Atropine may be given for hypersalivation.

Diazepam or pentobarbitone may be used to control twitching, fasciculation or convulsions.

Diazepam dose: 0.5 mg/kg body weight i.v. repeated every 10 minutes up to three times if needed. Pentobarbitone dose: 3–15 mg/kg body weight by slow intravenous infusion.

Care should be taken to maintain hydration and body temperature. If temperature rises due to muscle fasciculation cerebral oedema may result, which can lead to continued convulsions.

Fatty foods should not be given because these will enhance absorption.

References and further reading

VPIS (London) past cases up to 97/76977 (permethrin), 97/124304 (pyrethroids).

Nicholson SS (1995). Toxicity of insecticides and skin care products of botanical origin. *Veterinary Dermatology* **6(3)**, 139–143.

Valentine WM (1990). Pyrethrin and pyrethroid insecticides. *Veterinary Clinics of North America: Small Animal Practice* **20(2)**, 375–382.

Rhododendron and related plant species

The plant

Common names are azalea and rhododendron. Rhododendron and related species are usually hardy, evergreen or deciduous shrubs and trees. They are found outdoors and as house and conservatory plants and may grow to heights of approximately 5 metres. They are not native to the UK. Since their introduction as garden shrubs, they have become naturalised in many places, often forming dense thickets in the countryside.

The most widely naturalised species, *Rhododendron ponticum* is a large, branched shrub, often with a well-developed trunk. *Rhododendron ponticum* is found in woodlands and heaths, on acid, peaty, or sandy soils.

Leaves are elliptical, pointed, leathery, usually shiny, dark green above, paler beneath and hairless. Flowers are either bell- or funnel-shaped, approximately 5 cm in length, and are borne in conspicuous rounded clusters at the end of branches or occasionally arising from the side shoots. Colours range from white through red, pink and purple. The fruit is a dry, oblong capsule.

Occurrence of poisoning incidences

Since the launch of the VPIS, the centre in London has received a number of enquiries each year regarding exposure to rhododendron. Some of these enquiries concern livestock but several also involve dogs. No fatal cases in dogs have been reported, although all canine cases reported to the VPIS have been symptomatic.

A case from the literature describes how five dogs developed lethargy and ataxia after walking through a wood where shredded *Rhododendron ponticum* was present. Some of the animals developed lassitude, yawning, and head rubbing. One animal also presented some difficulty in picking up food, followed by gaseous efflux from the stomach, but no vomiting. There was no ingestion, only paw and muzzle contact. Three of the dogs were under care for other conditions, so no reliable conclusion can be drawn (Frape and Ward, 1993).

Toxicity

Poisonings usually occur in gardens or in woodland areas, often when the animals are exercising. Rhododendron species are highly toxic to all animals and clinical effects are similar for all species. All parts of the plant are toxic, including the nectar.

Mechanism of toxicity

Rhododendron species contain several diterpene resinoids called grayano-toxins. These are found in the nectar, leaves, and stems. Eighteen grayanotoxins have been isolated from species in the Ericaceae family. The main toxin in rhododendron species is grayanotoxin I, also known as rhodotoxin, acetylandromedol or andromedotoxin.

Grayanotoxins bind to receptors of the open and closed sodium channel of cell membranes. Binding results in a modified sodium channel that undergoes slow opening. The activated cells maintain a persistent excitation and depolarisation. Excitable cells in the nerves and muscle are maintained in a state of depolarisation at which time the entry of calcium into the cell is made. The sodium-channel effects of grayanotoxins account for the severe weakness, hypotension, dyspnoea, cardiac and neurological signs observed with rhododendron toxicity.

Kinetics and metabolism

Limited information is available on the kinetics of grayanotoxins. Experimental work in mice and rats indicate that grayanotoxins are rapidly metabolised and excreted.

Clinical effects

Clinical effects have a rapid onset usually occurring within 20 minutes to 2 hours. Initially, gastrointestinal signs predominate. The rapid development of these gastrointestinal effects may discourage significant ingestions. Clinical effects rarely last longer than 24 hours, presumably because grayanotoxins are rapidly eliminated.

Clinical signs seen in cases of rhododendron poisoning are similar for all animal species. These include salivation, vomiting, diarrhoea, inappetence, abdominal tenderness, trembling, staggering, lethargy, weakness, brady-cardia, hypotension and exhaustion.

Fatal cases are very rare in dogs, but would occur within a few hours of ingestion due to respiratory failure.

Post-mortem findings

Findings are usually non-specific. Plant fragments in the stomach are common in livestock who have ingested parts of the plant. Haemorrhagic enteritis would be anticipated.

Treatment

If the animal has not vomited and is presented to surgery within 2 hours of the ingestion then use of emesis and absorbents is recommended. Gastric lavage is probably unnecessary.

Emetics:

(a) Apomorphine	Dose:	0.05 mg/kg body weight i.v. or i.m.; 0.1 mg/kg body weight s.c.
(b) Xylazine	Dose:	0.2 mg/kg body weight i.v.; 0.5–1 mg/kg body weight i.m. or s.c.
(c) Ipecacuanha	Dose:	1–2 ml/kg body weight (maximum 20 ml) orally
(d) Soda crystal.		

Adsorbents:

| (a) Activated charcoal | Dose: | 2 g/kg body weight orally |
| (b) BCK granules® | Dose: | 6–18 g orally two or three times daily. |

Management thereafter is symptomatic and supportive, as there is no specific antidote. A minimum observation period of 6 hours post-ingestion is recommended. The animal should be kept well hydrated.

Atropine is a partial antagonist of the cardiac effects of grayanotoxins and may be considered if the animal develops severe bradycardia. Atropine dose: 30–100 μg/kg body weight s.c. or i.m.; 20 μg/kg body weight i.v.

Investigative

There are no clinically useful toxicological tests.

References and further reading

VPIS (London) past cases up to 97/124588.

Frape D and Ward A (1993). Suspected rhododendron poisoning in dogs. *Veterinary Record* **132**, 515–516.

Hikino H *et al.* (1979). Subchronic toxicity of ericaceous toxins and rhododendron leaves. *Chemical and Pharmaceutical Bulletin* **27**, 874–879.

Mayer S (1991). Rhododendron. *In Practice* **13(6)**, 222.

Rose F (1991). *The Wild Flower Key*. Frederick Warne, pp. 276–277.

Seyama I and Narahasi T (1981). Modulation of sodium channels of squid nerve membranes by grayanotoxin I. *Journal of Pharmacology and Experimental Therapeutics* **219(3)**, 614–624.

Sutlupinar N *et al.* (1993). Poisoning by toxic honey in turkey. *Archives of Toxicology* **67(2)**, 148–150.

Rowan / *Sorbus aucuparia*

The plant

The common name is Rowan or Mountain ash. The plant belongs to the Rosaceae family.

This deciduous tree is commonly found throughout the UK. The leaves may be up to 30 cm long and occur in pairs off the mid-rib. It flowers from May to June with a creamy blossom. The berries are orange-red, or sometimes yellow, and develop and ripen from August onwards, remaining on the plant to December. The berries contain up to three light-coloured seeds.

Occurrence of poisoning incidences

Since the launch of the VPIS, the centre in London has received a small number of enquiries each year regarding ingestion of Rowan by dogs. Most cases remain asymptomatic. Those with clinical effects displayed mild gastrointestinal effects only.

Toxicity

This plant is considered of low toxicity.

Mechanism of toxicity

The plant contains the cyanogenic glycoside amygdalin, and also parascorbic acid, which is irritant to mucous membranes. They are present in very low concentrations and therefore rarely cause more than gastrointestinal effects.

Clinical effects

Vomiting, diarrhoea, and salivation are the only effects reported in past VPIS cases.

Treatment

Gastric decontamination using gastric lavage, emesis or adsorbents is not necessary unless huge amounts of plant material have been ingested.

Management should otherwise be supportive, particularly ensuring that the animal is well hydrated.

Reference

VPIS (London) past cases up to 97/89921.

Salbutamol

Type of product

Salbutamol is a selective β_2-adrenoceptor agonist with effects on both smooth and skeletal muscle. It has use in human medicine as a bronchodilator for use in patients with asthma, chronic bronchitis, emphysema or other chronic airway obstruction. It also has a use in management of premature labour.

Presentation

Salbutamol is available in many forms in the UK. It is a prescription-only medicine.

Tablets are usually of 2 mg, 4 mg or 8 mg strength and syrup preparations of 2 mg/5 ml are available. Respirator solution and solutions for nebulisers commonly have strengths of 5 mg/ml and either 1 mg/ml or 2 mg/ml, respectively. Disks and capsules for inhalers are usually of 200 μg or 400 μg strength.

Note: In the USA, salbutamol is called albuterol.

Occurrence of poisoning incidences

Since the launch of the VPIS in 1992, enquiries to the VPIS London centre about salbutamol have been common, representing approximately 1.1% of the annual total. Over 90% of these enquiries involve canine cases, with the chewing of the inhalers being the most common circumstance. Fatalities have been very few, but many animals have displayed signs of intoxication.

Recommended dosage

In the UK, the drug is supplied for use in humans only.

Toxicity

Salbutamol toxicity usually causes rapid onset of clinical effects, which are generally mild and short-lived. All but two cases reported to VPISLn have recovered without sequelae.

In the experience of the VPISLn:

- 3.2 mg/kg body weight, ingested as tablets, caused severe tachycardia and tremors, requiring sedation but with complete recovery within 24 hours (VPISLn case 92/55369).

- 2.8 mg/kg body weight, ingested as tablets, caused tachycardia, periorbital oedema, dilated pupils, and pyrexia, which resolved over 24 hours (VPISLn case 93/12091).
- Two cases of ingestion of a single inhaler in dogs resulted in fatality. The dogs weighed 25 kg and 40 kg. The lighter one became weak, tachypnoeic, tachycardic and cyanosed, whilst the other became very tachycardic and showed evidence of poor peripheral circulation. Both animals died of shock (VPISLn cases 97/37032 and 97/130464).

Mechanism of toxicity

The clinical effects in poisoning cases can be seen to be a direct result of the β_2-agonist activity of the drug. These would include relaxation of smooth muscle, which is probably mediated via the adenyl cyclase-cyclic adenosine monophosphate system.

Clinical effects

Clinical effects have an onset between 30 minutes and 8 hours post-exposure, but commonly within 4 hours. Recovery is usually within 8–24 hours. Rarely, effects may persist for 36–48 hours.

Tachycardia and hyperpnoea are the most common features of salbutamol poisoning in dogs. Other reported effects include incoordination, lethargy, restlessness, thirst, peripheral vasodilation, tremor, muscle weakness, twitching, hypokalaemia, depression and anxiety. Effects more rarely observed are vomiting, pyrexia, dilated pupils and periorbital oedema. Temporary spastic paralysis has been observed in two VPISLn cases (87/42873 and 94/11832). In the two fatal cases reported to the VPISLn, the animals collapsed and went into shock.

Treatment

Treatment is necessary if a dose greater than 1 mg/kg has been exceeded.

If within 2 hours of ingestion, induce vomiting or perform gastric lavage, and then administer adsorbents.

Emetics:

(a) Apomorphine	Dose:	0.05 mg/kg body weight i.v. or i.m.; 0.1 mg/kg body weight s.c.
(b) Xylazine	Dose:	0.2 mg/kg body weight i.v.; 0.5–1 mg/kg body weight i.m. or s.c.
(c) Ipecacuanha	Dose:	1–2 ml/kg body weight (maximum 20 ml) orally
(d) Soda crystal.		

Adsorbents:

(a) Activated charcoal	Dose:	2 g/kg body weight orally
(b) BCK granules®	Dose:	6–18 g orally two or three times daily.

Treatment thereafter is largely supportive. Observation is recommended for at least 4 hours post-ingestion. If the animal does develop clinical effects then electrolytes, especially potassium, should be checked and corrected where possible.

Diazepam or acepromazine may be given for sedative or anticonvulsant purposes. Where adsorbents have been administered then use parenteral routes. Diazepam dose: 0.5 mg/kg body weight i.v. repeated every 10 minutes up to three times if needed. Acepromazine dose: 1–3 mg/kg body weight orally; 0.03–0.1 mg/kg body weight i.m., or s.c.; 0.03 mg/kg body weight by slow i.v. injection.

Propranolol or atenolol may be given for severe or prolonged tachycardia. Where adsorbents have been administered then use parenteral routes and doses. Propranolol dose: 0.02–0.15 mg/kg body weight i.v. over 2–3 minutes; 0.2–1.0 mg/kg body weight orally two to three times daily. Atenolol dose: 0.1–1 mg/kg body weight orally twice daily.

References

VPIS (London) past cases up to 97/130464.

Owens JG and Dorman DC (1997). Drug poisoning in small animals. *Veterinary Medicine* **92(2)**, 149–156.

Salt / sodium chloride

Type of product

Sodium chloride is widely available and has many uses. Possible sources include modelling dough, cooking salt, bottle sterilising fluids, water softeners, dishwasher salt, sea water and salt used to de-ice roads in winter.

Presentation

It occurs as a white crystalline powder or colourless cuboidal crystals. One gram of sodium chloride contains 17.2 mmol of sodium. One teaspoon of sodium chloride weighs about 7.25 g (125 mmol); a tablespoon weighs 14.5–21.75 g, equivalent to 250–375 mmol.

A typical recipe for homemade modelling dough is 100 g salt, 200 g flour and about 100 ml water. Dough weighing 1 g contains approximately 250 mg of salt when wet and approximately 300 mg when dried.

Occurrence of poisoning incidences

Enquiries to the VPIS regarding salt ingestion are infrequent. However, when cases do arise they generally involve dogs with severe clinical effects and fatal outcomes are common. The most common sources of sodium chloride in these canine cases is commercially available modelling dough for small children. Three fatal cases involving such products have been reported to the VPIS London centre.

Toxicity

According to the literature:

- Dogs are reported to be able to ingest 4 g/kg body weight a day without adverse effect.
- 3.7 g/kg body weight has been quoted as the lethal dose for dogs.

In the experience of the VPISLn:

- Mortality is high.
- Ingestion of an estimated 180 g modelling dough by a 22 kg Border Collie resulted in severe clinical effects in a dog who then deteriorated, despite aggressive management and required euthanasia (VPISLn case 94/53482).

Mechanism of toxicity

Sodium contributes to about 90% of the osmolality of the extracellular fluid and an increase in sodium will thus increase the plasma omolality. This results in the extracellular fluid becoming hypertonic and water moving from the intracellular to the extracellular space. The net result is cellular dehydration and vascular overload. In the CNS, this will cause vascular stasis, thrombosis, brain shrinkage and shearing of intracerebral vessels with subsequent haemorrhage.

The normal range of sodium in dogs is 137–149 mmol/L. In a reported fatal case of ingestion of salt in a dog there was continued absorption of salt from the gut due to crystallisation of the large quantity ingested. At post-mortem there was at least 20 g of sodium chloride found in the stomach (Khanna *et al.*, 1997).

Case reports

A 20 kg 8-year-old male Airedale terrier presented at a clinic with a 45-minute history of continuous convulsions. The dog had ingested a salt–flour figurine (about 100 g) 36 hours prior to presentation. The dog had vomited three times within 12 hours of ingestion and became progressively more polydipsic and polyuric. The owner had removed the dog's drinking water after 24 hours because it had been urinating every 10–15 minutes. Polyuria continued for 7 hours during which time he ingested an unknown additional quantity of uncooked salt–flour mixture. Within 1 hour of this second ingestion the dog developed generalised fine-muscular fascicula-tion, which rapidly progressed to convulsions. On presentation no details of the salt–flour ingestion were given by the owner. On examination the animal was found to be an estimated 8% dehydrated, unresponsive to painful stimuli and pyrexic. It had an elevated respiratory rate and irregular heart rhythm, weak pulse, tachycardia (240 beats/minute) with a prolonged QT interval. The dog was given diazepam and dexamethasone and started on intravenous fluids. Laboratory analysis revealed severe hypernatraemia (211 mmol/L), hyperchloraemia (180 mmol/L) and metabolic acidosis (pH 7.1.35). Ingestion of the salt–flour mixture was disclosed on discussion with the owners. The intravenous fluids were changed to dextrose and sodium bicarbonate and frusemide were given. Convulsions recurred despite the diazepam infusion and phenobarbitone was added. Cooling measures were undertaken but the dog remained unresponsive for 4 hours. The pulse rate fell to 160 beats/minute and the body temperature decreased. The sodium and chloride concentrations initially decreased after 2 hours but increased again at 4 hours. Intravenous fluids were increased and sodium bicarbonate discontinued. The acidosis worsened after changing to dextrose, the respiratory rate remained elevated and the dog subsequently suffered respiratory arrest. Manual ventilation was followed by cardiac arrest. Resuscitation was discontinued. The sodium concentration was 210 mmol/L, chloride 167 mmol/L, pH 6.72.

Post-mortem examination revealed 1 litre of putty-like, grey-white material and watery fluid in the stomach. There was haemorrhage in the stomach and the proximal two-thirds of the small intestine. Patchy areas of haemorrhage were observed in the colon. Acute renal and hepatic necrosis was documented and there was diffuse white-matter vacuolation in the brain. Analysis of the liquid portion of the stomach contents showed that it contained at least 20 g of sodium chloride (Khanna *et al.*, 1997).

A Golden Retriever of unknown age developed vomiting initially and then diarrhoea 12 hours after ingesting two tubs of Playstuff®, a children's modelling dough. Acute renal failure developed 3 days later and the dog died 4 days post-ingestion. The treating veterinarian considered that the over-zealous rehydration in this case probably contributed to the fatal outcome of the case (VPISLn case 94/3680).

A 5-year-old female Border Collie (22 kg) was fed Funstuff® and Play Doh® by a child during a tea party. The dog developed anorexia about 24 hours later and repeated vomiting about 24 hours after that. The dog presented to surgery with dehydration about 3 days after onset of vomiting. It was treated with antibiotics, anti-inflammatories and anti-emetics but did not improve. Intensive i.v. fluid therapy was commenced. Renal failure was evident, with raised urea and creatinine concentrations. The dog gradually deteriorated and was euthanased 9 days after ingestion (VPISLn case 94/53482).

Clinical effects

These are vomiting, diarrhoea, lethargy, tremor, thirst and dehydration (the degree of dehydration may be underestimated because the vascular volume is maintained).

In severe cases, muscular rigidity, convulsions, coma and renal failure may occur. Shock may occur due to severe intracellular fluid loss. Hyperchloraemia and mixed metabolic and respiratory acidosis has been reported.

At post-mortem, there may be renal congestion and inflammation and congestion of the gastrointestinal tract.

Treatment

Since vomiting is common and usually profuse, emesis is not recommended. It may also exacerbate any dehydration. Gastric lavage following a large ingestion of sodium chloride may enhance absorption through dissolution and although surgical removal may be considered in severe cases, the animal may be too unwell to tolerate anaesthesia. Adsorbents are not useful.

The sodium concentration, the chloride concentration and renal function should be monitored. Symptomatic and supportive care are required and anti-emetics may be given if vomiting is excessive. Anticonvulsants may be required in severe cases.

Note: The aim of therapy is to lower the sodium concentration slowly. Rapid reduction may lead to cerebral oedema.

In mild cases, the animal should be allowed to drink small amounts of fresh water at frequent intervals.

In more severe cases, parenteral fluids will be required. These should contain low quantities of sodium, e.g. 5% dextrose or 2.5% dextrose in 0.45% saline. These fluids should be administered with care and recovery may take several days.

References and further reading

VPIS (London) past cases up to 97/64523.

Duncan A (1992). Poison – salt. *In Practice* **14(5)**, 252.

Khanna C, Boermans HJ and Wilcock B (1997). Fatal hypernatremia in a dog from salt ingestion. *Journal of the American Animal Hospital Association* **33**, 113–117.

Selective serotonin re-uptake inhibitor antidepressants

Type of product

These are antidepressant drugs for human use. One of the drugs in this group, fluoxetine, has been proposed for use in small animals for management of stereotypies, anxiety, aggression and 'depression'.

Presentation

They are available in tablet and/or capsule preparations of various strengths:

Citalopram	10 mg, 20 mg
Fluoxetine	20 mg, 60 mg
Fluvoxamine	50 mg, 100 mg
Paroxetine	20 mg, 30 mg
Sertraline	50 mg, 100 mg

Fluoxetine and paroxetine are also available in liquid preparations at strengths of 20 mg/5 ml and 10 mg/5 ml, respectively.

Occurrence of poisoning incidences

Since the launch of the VPIS in 1992, an increasing number of enquiries have been handled each year regarding SSRI antidepressant ingestion by dogs. In 1997 and 1998 over 20 enquiries per annum were received. This probably reflects increasing use by humans and therefore increased availability. Few cases have displayed clinical effects and no fatal cases have been reported.

Recommended dosage

Fluoxetine: 1 mg/kg body weight orally once daily for stereotypies, aggression, anxiety, and depression.

Toxicity

These drugs appear to be of low toxicity.

According to the literature:

Citalopram

- 20–25 mg/kg body weight given either intravenously or orally resulted in convulsions.

- Lower doses caused drowsiness, restlessness, anxiety, aggression and tachycardia.

Fluoxetine

- In LD_{50} studies in dogs no deaths were reported for a dose in excess of 100 mg/kg body weight.
- Dogs given 20 mg/kg/day for 90 days had mild anorexia, transient dilated pupils, vomiting, fine tremor and loose, mucoid faeces. With doses of 50 mg/kg for 11 months, one dog died after 50 days due to convulsions. In addition to the effects seen with the lower dose, the animals also had increased salivation.

Fluvoxamine

- The LD_{50} in dogs is greater than 450 mg/kg body weight.
- Clinical effects observed in these studies included vomiting, dilated pupils, ataxia, convulsions and bradypnoea.

In the experience of the VPISLn:

Fluoxetine

- Doses as high as 14 mg/kg body weight have resulted in no clinical effects.

Paroxetine

- A Golden Retriever became drowsy and developed unspecified ECG abnormalities after ingestion of 3 mg/kg body weight (VPISLn case 95/51696).
- A Yorkshire terrier developed inappetence, laboured breathing and 'dullness' after ingesting 8 mg/kg body weight (VPISLn case 95/122877).
- In other cases, doses between 2.35 and 7.5 mg/kg body weight produced no clinical effects.

Sertraline

- Doses between 12 and 24 mg/kg body weight resulted in no clinical effects.

Kinetics and metabolism

The drugs appear to be rapidly absorbed. In clinical trials for fluvoxamine in dogs, the peak plasma levels were reached between 2 and 4 hours post-ingestion.

The plasma half-life in dogs after 15 doses of 5–10 mg/kg was 1 day for fluoxetine and 2.1–5.4 days for the primary amine metabolite.

There is evidence to suggest that these drugs undergo some enterohepatic recirculation in dogs.

Clinical effects

Clinical effects usually occur within 4 hours of ingestion.

Drowsiness, ataxia, and inappetence are reported in VPISLn cases. Unspecified ECG abnormalities lasting 2–3 days have been reported.

Other possible effects include convulsions with high doses, restlessness, anxiety, aggression, tachycardia, dilated pupils, vomiting, bradypnoea, fine tremor and loose, mucoid faeces.

Treatment

Treatment is recommended if more than 10 mg/kg body weight has been ingested for all these drugs except paroxetine, where treatment is recommended if more than 5 mg/kg body weight has been eaten.

If within 2 hours of ingestion and if the animal is not drowsy, induce vomiting or perform gastric lavage. Adsorbents should then be given.

Emetics:

(a)	Apomorphine	Dose:	0.05 mg/kg body weight i.v. or i.m.; 0.1 mg/kg body weight s.c.
(b)	Xylazine	Dose:	0.2 mg/kg body weight i.v.; 0.5–1 mg/kg body weight i.m. or s.c.
(c)	Ipecacuanha	Dose:	1–2 ml/kg body weight (maximum 20 ml) orally
(d)	Soda crystal.		

Adsorbents:

(a)	Activated charcoal	Dose:	2 g/kg body weight orally
(b)	BCK granules®	Dose:	6–18 g orally.

Management is otherwise supportive. Diazepam may be given for convulsions if needed. Diazepam dose: 0.5 mg/kg body weight i.v. repeated every 10 minutes up to three times if needed. A 6-hour minimum observation period is recommended.

Reference

VPIS (London) past cases up to 97/84889.

Sex hormones

Type of product

Sex hormones are used in a variety of disorders in veterinary medicine. Oestradiol is used for the provision of short-term oestrogen therapy for the treatment of misalliance, hypogonadal obesity and hormone urinary incontinence in bitches and anal adenomata, excess libido and prostatic hyperplasia in the male. The progestagen, proligesterone is used for the control of oestrus in bitches.

Sex hormones are widely used in human medicine for oral contraception and hormone replacement therapy (HRT).

Presentation

Injectable preparations are available for veterinary use but numerous tablet formulations are available for oral contraception in humans. Transdermal patches, gels, creams and pessaries are also used in human medicine for hormone replacement therapy. Oral contraceptives may contain oestrogens and progesterone or progesterone only. HRT formulations may contain oestrogen and/or progesterone.

Occurrence of poisoning incidences

Since the launch of the VPIS in 1992, the London centre has received between 20 and 70 enquiries per annum regarding ingestion of hormonal preparations by dogs and cats. Most of these involved preparations intended for human use. Almost all cases remained asymptomatic. Those rare cases with clinical effects displayed mild gastrointestinal effects only.

Most animals were exposed to human preparations, particularly oral contraceptives and hormone replacement therapy (HRT).

Recommended dosage

This varies, depending on the specific drug and the indication.

Toxicity

These drugs are considered of low toxicity in acute overdose.

Clinical effects

Usually there are no effects from ingestion of these products but vomiting and diarrhoea may occur. Progesterone-containing preparations may disrupt oestrus in bitches.

Treatment

No treatment is necessary, even for very substantial ingestions.

Reference

VPIS (London) past cases up to 98/165110.

Terfenadine

Type of product

Terfenadine is an antihistamine used for the symptomatic relief of hypersensitivity reactions such as rhinitis and urticaria in human medicine. It is not used in veterinary medicine.

Presentation

Terfenadine is available in the UK in both tablet and liquid preparations. Tablet strengths are usually 60 or 120 mg and the liquid suspensions of 30 mg/5 ml strength.

Occurrence of poisoning incidences

Since the launch of the VPIS in 1992, there have been between five and 10 enquiries per annum regarding terfenadine exposure in dogs. No cases have had a fatal outcome, though some animals have exhibited severe clinical effects.

Recommended dosage

In the UK, the drug is supplied for use in humans only.

Toxicity

According to the literature:

- In a case review study, doses causing clinical effects in dogs ranged from 6.6 to 557 mg/kg body weight.
- Wide variety in toxic doses may be due to individual variation or variation in susceptibility due to differences in breed or age.
- Pre-clinical studies in dogs reported no clinical effects in dogs fed 30 mg/kg body weight for 2 years.
- Doses of 100 mg/kg body weight resulted in ataxia, trembling, rigidity, weakness, disorientation and convulsions in three out of eight study dogs after 2–3 weeks of treatment. In these cases, no ECG changes were apparent.
- Doses of 150 mg/kg body weight consistently resulted in vomiting.

In the experience of the VPISLn:

- It is considered to have a relatively low toxicity.
- Doses of up to 46 mg/kg body weight in a variety of breeds resulted in no visible clinical effects.

- 24 mg/kg body weight ingested by a collie resulted in hyperaesthesia, ataxia, congested mucous membranes, tachycardia, tachypnoea, dilated pupils and hyperthermia. Emesis was attempted without success, and the animal was given diazepam and acepromazine. With supportive care the animal made a slow recovery (VPISLn case 91/9999).
- 48 mg/kg body weight in a Yorkshire Terrier resulted in weakness, pale mucous membranes, drowsiness, twitching and fitting. The animal made a slow recovery with supportive care (VPISLn case 97/119316).
- 60 mg/kg body weight in a Labrador resulted in tremors, incoordination and apparent blindness. Emesis was induced, and the animal given intravenous fluid support and diazepam and made a slow recovery (VPISLn case 96/183192).
- No fatal cases reported.

Mechanism of toxicity

Terfenadine is a butyrophenone derivative. Like many antihistamines it acts by reversibly and competitively blocking the action of histamine at the receptor site, thereby reducing the pharmacological action. At high doses the binding becomes irreversible.

In overdose, antihistamines cause anticholinergic effects and CNS depression or stimulation. The mechanism of the CNS effects is largely unknown, although terfenadine causes minimal CNS effects in therapy since it does not readily cross the blood–brain barrier. In dogs, EEG changes have been observed with doses of 30 mg/kg and it is assumed at such doses the blood–brain barrier may be crossed.

Kinetics and metabolism

Peak plasma concentrations in dogs given terfenadine on an empty stomach was at 3 hours; the half-life of the major metabolite (the carboxylic acid derivative) was 17 hours. Terfenadine is metabolised in the liver and excreted in the urine. High doses may result in prolonged elimination.

Clinical effects

The onset of clinical effects is usually relatively rapid and within 4–6 hours. Complete recovery appears to be protracted in animals who develop clinical signs.

Commonly reported effects are dry mucous membranes or salivation, vomiting, dilated pupils, ataxia, tachycardia, tachypnoea and hypotension.

Occasionally reported effects include weakness, lethargy, apparent hallucinations, hyperthermia, agitation, hyperaesthesia and anxiety. Rarely reported effects include disorientation, polydipsia, convulsions, rigidity and polyuria.

Treatment

Treatment is recommended if more than 25 mg/kg body weight has been ingested.

If within 2 hours of ingestion induce vomiting, after ensuring that there is an adequate swallowing reflex, and then administer adsorbents.

Where the swallowing reflex is reduced or absent, give adsorbents only.

Emetics:

(a) Apomorphine   Dose: 0.05 mg/kg body weight i.v. or i.m.; 0.1 mg/kg body weight s.c.

(b) Xylazine   Dose: 0.2 mg/kg body weight i.v.; 0.5–1 mg/kg body weight i.m. or s.c.

(c) Ipecacuanha   Dose: 1–2 ml/kg body weight (maximum 20 ml) orally

(d) Soda crystal.

Adsorbents:

(a) Activated charcoal   Dose: 2 g/kg body weight orally

(b) BCK granules®   Dose: 6–18 g orally two or three times daily.

Treatment thereafter is largely supportive, with particular care to ensure adequate hydration, normal body temperature and monitoring of blood pressure and pulse. Observation for a minimum period of 4 hours is advocated.

Sedation may be required for animals that appear to hallucinate or fit. Diazepam or acepromazine have been recommended for use in the past. Diazepam, however, should be used with caution as antihistamines such as terfenadine are known to potentiate the depressant effects of benzodiazepines. Diazepam dose: 0.5 mg/kg body weight i.v. repeated every 10 minutes up to three times if needed. Acepromazine dose: 1–3 mg/kg body weight orally; 0.03–0.1 mg/kg body weight i.m., or s.c.; 0.03 mg/kg body weight by slow i.v. injection.

References and further reading

VPIS (London) past cases up to 97/119316.

Papich MG (1990). Toxicoses from over-the-counter human drugs. *Veterinary Clinics of North America: Small Animal Practice* **20(2)**, 431–451.

Otto CM and Greentree WF (1994). Terfenadine toxicosis in dogs. *Journal of the American Veterinary Medical Association* **205(7)**, 1004–1006.

Owens JG and Dorman DC (1997). Drug poisoning in small animals. *Veterinary Medicine* **92(2)**, 149–156.

Tricyclic antidepressants

Type of product

These are antidepressant drugs for human use. Tricyclic antidepressants are the most commonly prescribed type of antidepressants in the UK. They have a good safety profile in humans when used at recommended dosages but are toxic in overdose.

Some of these agents are used in veterinary medicine as anxiolytics and also in the management of separation problems, excessive grooming, feline urine spaying, acral lick dermatitis and compulsive stereotypic behaviours. They have also rarely been used to treat canine narcoleptic hypersomnia.

Presentation

They are available in tablet or capsule preparations of various strengths for each drug. Maximum dose for tablets or capsules available for all included drugs is 75 mg.

Some of the drugs are available in syrup preparations: amitriptyline, clomipramine and imipramine at 25 mg/5 ml strength and lofepramine at 70 mg/5 ml strength.

Substances included are **amitriptyline, clomipramine, dothiepin, doxepin, imipramine, lofepramine, nortriptyline, protriptyline, and trimipramine.**

Occurrence of poisoning incidences

Since the launch of the VPIS in 1992, between five and 15 enquiries have been received per annum concerning tricyclic antidepressant ingestion by dogs. Some 10% have exhibited some clinical effects, but there have been no fatal outcomes reported.

Recommended dosage

Amitriptyline:	1–2 mg/kg body weight given orally daily in divided doses for anxiety, separation problems and excessive grooming.
Clomipramine:	1–3 mg/kg body weight given orally daily for anxiety, separation problems, and stereotypies.
Doxepin:	0.5–1 mg/kg body weight given orally daily for compulsive stereotypic behaviour.

Toxicity

According to the literature:

- 100 mg/kg body weight is the lowest published lethal oral dose of imipramine in dogs.
- Intravenous administration of 20 mg/kg body weight of various tricyclic antidepressants caused death within 50 minutes of injection.
- Canine ingestion of doses greater than 15 mg/kg body weight are anticipated to result in severe toxicity or fatality.

In the experience of the VPISLn:

- 25 mg of amitriptyline given to a German Shepherd dog resulted in excitability, hyperventilation, and tachycardia. The animal recovered with supportive care only.
- 35 mg/kg body weight given to a terrier mongrel resulted in no clinical effects.
- 450 mg of dothiepin ingested by a West Highland terrier resulted in dilated pupils, vocalising, hyperventilation, hyperaesthesia and fitting. The animal was given activated charcoal and diazepam and made a gradual recovery over 12 hours (VPISLn case 91/5473).

Mechanism of toxicity

Tricyclic antidepressants are thought to act by blocking the re-uptake of noradrenaline and 5-hydroxytryptamine (5-HT) in the CNS. Additionally, they also block the parasympathetic nervous system and the peripheral re-uptake of noradrenaline and also have a membrane-stabilising effect (quinidine-like) on the myocardium mediated by disruption of the sodium/potassium pump.

A combination of these effects is also responsible for the toxic effects. The blockage of the parasympathetic nervous system and the noradrenaline re-uptake results in anticholinergic signs such as tachycardia, dilated pupils, urine retention, gastric stasis, dry mucous membranes, tremors and convulsions. The effects of the membrane stabilising effect is most pronounced on the myocardium where the refractory period increases and conduction velocity decreases. This is reflected on the ECG where the PR, QT and QRS intervals and complex increase in duration. Ventricular arrhythmias are the clinical result.

Kinetics and metabolism

The tricyclic antidepressants are rapidly absorbed from the gastrointestinal tract, bind to plasma proteins and have a high volume of distribution. Owing to their anticholinergic action, gastric emptying may be delayed and therefore at higher doses more drug may be absorbed. The drugs also undergo enterohepatic re-circulation.

The drugs are metabolised in the liver and undergo demethylation and hydroxylation and then glucuronide conjugation. Excretion is via the kidney.

Clinical effects

Clinical effects usually occur within 4 hours.

Excitability, vomiting, ataxia, lethargy, and tremors are common. Dilated pupils, dry mucous membranes, urine retention, hypotension, and tachycardia are occasionally reported.

In severe cases the animal may become very drowsy or comatose, and may also develop respiratory depression, convulsions and ventricular arrhythmias.

Prolongation of the PR, QT and QRS intervals and complex may be evident on the ECG, and the animal may develop ventricular arrhythmias.

The animal may also develop metabolic acidosis and hypokalaemia.

Treatment

Treatment is recommended if more than 5 mg/kg body weight has been ingested.

If within 2 hours of ingestion and if the animal is not drowsy, induce vomiting. Alternatively, gastric lavage may be performed.

Adsorbents should then be given. Some authors suggest that repeated doses of adsorbents may be of benefit, although there is some evidence to suggest limited efficacy as only a small percentage undergoes enterohepatic re-circulation.

Emetics:

(a) Apomorphine	Dose:	0.05 mg/kg body weight i.v. or i.m.; 0.1 mg/kg body weight s.c.
(b) Xylazine	Dose:	0.2 mg/kg body weight i.v.; 0.5–1 mg/kg body weight i.m. or s.c.
(c) Ipecacuanha	Dose:	1–2 ml/kg body weight (maximum 20 ml) orally
(d) Soda crystal.		

Adsorbents:

(a) Activated charcoal	Dose:	2 g/kg body weight orally
(b) BCK granules®	Dose:	6–18 g orally.

These doses may be repeated at 2–3 hourly intervals until the adsorbent appears in the stools if felt necessary or if ingested dose was very large.

Animals need close observation for a minimum of 9 hours. Management is largely symptomatic and supportive. However, particular care should be taken to ensure adequate hydration.

Intravenous fluid support may be required to maintain the blood pressure.

Where possible electrolytes, especially potassium, and blood gases should be monitored and corrected where appropriate.

If the animal develops severe tremors or convulsions then diazepam may be given. Diazepam dose: 0.5 mg/kg body weight i.v. repeated every 10 minutes up to three times if needed. Where respiratory depression becomes severe, ventilation may be considered.

Where possible, the ECG should be monitored. If there is evidence of tachycardia and particularly cardiac conduction abnormalities, such as a widened QRS, then intravenous sodium bicarbonate should be administered to maintain arterial pH at approximately 7.5. Additionally, potassium should be supplemented, where necessary, to ensure plasma levels are within the normal range.

Sodium bicarbonate dose: 2–3 mmol/kg body weight i.v. over 15–30 minutes (approximately equivalent to 15–20 ml/kg body weight of a 1.24% solution).

References and further reading

VPIS (London) past cases up to 97/65219.

Johnson LR (1990). Tricyclic antidepressant toxicosis. *Veterinary Clinics of North America: Small Animal Practice* **20(2)**, 393–403.

Vipera berus berus / European adder

The snake

The European adder, *Vipera berus berus* (a member of the family Viperidae) is the only venomous snake native to the UK. It is also found across northern Europe, into the Arctic Circle, and Asia. It is a true viper, some 50–60 cm in length at maturity, varying in colour from pale grey to dark brown in the male and from olive green/yellowish-brown to reddish-brown in the female. It is distinguishable from the two other snakes native to Britain, the grass snake (*Natrix natrix*) and the smooth snake (*Coronella austriaca*), by a black/brown dorsal zig-zag patterning and a V-shaped marking on the head. However, in darker coloured male specimens this patterning may not be obvious. Another distinguishing feature is the eye of the adder, which is elliptical with a typical viperid vertical slit, as compared with the round-shaped eyes of the grass and smooth snakes. The adder is most commonly found on dry, sandy heaths, sand dunes, rocky hillsides, moorlands and woodland edges.

The adder generally only bites when provoked. Bites rarely occur during the winter when the snake is in hibernation but are frequent during the summer months. Not all bites result in envenomation.

Owing to increasing deliberate persecution, collection, and loss of its natural habitat, the adder is considered threatened throughout Europe. In 1991 a Statutory Instrument came into force to protect the snake in Britain (Wildlife and Countryside Act 1981 – Variation of Schedule Order 367).

Occurrence of poisoning incidences

Since 1992, the VPIS London centre has received a small number of enquiries every year regarding animal bites in animals, representing approximately 1% of the total enquiry number. Over 95% of these cases involve bites in dogs.

Toxicity

In domestic animals adder envenomations cause significant morbidity and high mortality, although the high mortality rate may be partly due to the difficulty experienced by many veterinarians in obtaining specific antivenom.

Mechanism of toxicity

The venom is a complex mixture of high molecular weight proteins, mainly proteases, peptide hydrolases, hyaluronidase and phospholipases, which are initially taken up into the lymphatics and then enter the systemic circulation. Hypovolaemia and local oedema result from an increase in vascular permeability, due initially to release of pharmacologically active substances such as histamine, serotonin, bradykinin and prostaglandins, and later due to direct result of venom on heart and blood vessels. Local haemorrhage is due to cytolytic and haemolytic factors.

Clinical effects

Reports indicate dogs are more likely to be bitten on the muzzle, the mouth, tongue or face. Bites to the feet or lower legs also occur. As dogs are reliant on panting as a means of control of body temperature, a bite to the face area is serious as the swelling that may occur following a bite may impair thermoregulation.

Localised painful swelling may occur within minutes of the bite or may be delayed for 30 minutes or more but is always present within 2 hours. Absence of swelling within 2 hours excludes envenomation.

The swelling will gradually spread and may be haemorrhagic. It may affect the animal's ability to eat and drink and to thermoregulate. There may be pale mucous membranes, bruising, salivation, vomiting, diarrhoea, dehydration, restlessness, drowsiness, depression, lethargy and lameness. The puncture wounds may be visible. Petechial haemorrhage of the gums has been seen in dogs bitten on the mouth. Necrosis is very rare.

Initially, tachycardia may be observed. Later there may be bradycardia, hypotension, collapse and shock. Pyrexia may be noted. Tremors and trembling are often noted and convulsions have been reported in one VPISLn case (85/32237). Some animals have developed chest and abdominal tenderness, and respiratory distress.

Severe coagulopathy may be noted in severe cases. The animal may also become anaemic, uraemic, thrombocytopaenic, hypoproteinaemic, and hypoalbuminaemic.

Death, usually associated with severe renal and hepatic dysfunction or failure, will usually occur in 5–7 days in dogs that receive no treatment.

Post-mortem findings

At post-mortem, lesions resulting from envenomation by the European Adder include haemorrhages, disseminated intravascular coagulation, hepatic necrosis and infarction. There may be haemorrhagic oedema at the bite site, pulmonary congestion, generalised haemolysis, icterus, myocardial degeneration, and petechial haemorrhages in the kidney cortex.

Treatment

Speed is essential. Ideally the affected animal needs to be kept as still and as quiet as possible. The bite site should be left alone and if the bite was to the leg, the affected limb should be immobilised if possible. Use of incisions, suction and tourniquets are not recommended as they may introduce infection, aggravate bleeding and restrict circulation.

Zagreb® **Antivenom** should be used in all cases where the bite was to the facial region and in all cases where the swelling is significant or has spread beyond the next major joint proximal to the bite. It should also be used if there is any indication of hypotension unresponsive to i.v. fluid therapy, any evidence of coagulopathy, or any ECG abnormality.

Dose: Some newer Zagreb® preparations are presented in 10 ml vials. The older vials were 5.5 ml volumes. Either 1 × 10 ml ampoule or 2 × 5.5 ml ampoules diluted in 2–3 volumes of isotonic saline administered by slow i.v. injection at a rate not exceeding 2 ml per minute is required. Alternatively, administer by i.v. infusion.

Clinical improvement should be seen rapidly, particularly if the antivenom is administered within 18 hours of the bite. If there is no clinical improvement within 2 hours of administration of the initial dose then the regimen may be repeated.

Note: The insert on the packaging indicates an i.m. route of administration. However, i.v. administration is perfectly safe and more likely to be effective.

The advice found in some sources suggesting that dogs require 10 vials of antivenom (or five of the new variety) is not correct. The normal prescribed dosage of two vials (or one of the new variety) is designed to counteract the venom of one snake bite. Excessive use of antivenom may result in the development of severe adverse reactions.

Adverse reactions to Zagreb®

These are very uncommon but if they occur (characterised by vomiting, fever, respiratory distress, bronchospasm occurring rapidly after antivenom administration) they can be minimised by giving the antivenom under the cover of adrenaline. Dose: 0.5–1.0 ml of a 1:1000 solution given s.c.

Supply of Zagreb®

In the experience of the VPISLn, veterinarians occasionally experience difficulties in obtaining Zagreb®. Usually the best source is the pharmacy or the Accident and Emergency Department of the local general hospital. The VPISLn may be able to advise on local supplies, and carries a small stock itself for dispatch in emergency cases. Cost of transport and antivenom will be to the veterinarian. The VPISLn is contactable on 020 7635 9195.

The current suppliers of Zagreb® in the UK are: Farillon Ltd, Ashton Road, Harold Hill, Romford, Essex RM3 8UE, UK (telephone: 01708 379000) and P & D

Pharmaceuticals, 38 Woolmer Way, Bordon, Hampshire GU35 9QF, UK (telephone: 01420 487501).

Other care

Generally, management is symptomatic and supportive. Observation is advised for any animal with clinical effects for a minimum period of 12 hours. Ensure adequate hydration, with i.v. fluids if needed, and monitor pulse, blood pressure, respiration and body temperature.

Metoclopramide may be given to control persistent vomiting. Dose: 0.5–1 mg/kg body weight i.m., s.c. or orally every 6–8 hours; 1–2 mg/kg i.v. over 24 hours as slow infusion.

Steroids (e.g. beclomethasone, dexamethasone, methylprednisolone) and anti-histamines (e.g. chlorpheniramine) have both been given in past cases to reduce swelling. In some cases, simple analgesia has been given.

Check for coagulopathy if there is any evidence of bleeding. Vitamin K_1 administration and blood transfusions have been necessary in some cases. Vitamin K_1 dose: 3–5 mg/kg body weight i.m. or s.c. daily in divided doses.

Diazepam may be given for convulsions. General anaesthesia may be considered if diazepam proves ineffective. Diazepam dose: 0.5 mg/kg body weight i.v. repeated every 10 minutes up to three times if needed.

In severe cases, monitor renal and hepatic function if possible.

References and further reading

VPIS (London) past cases up to 97/58208.

Bratberg B and Flesja K (1973). Intoxication in the dog by the European adder. *Nordisk Veterinaermedicin* **25**, 185 (in Norwegian).

Fowler ME (1992). Snakes and snakebite in Europe. In *Veterinary Zootoxicology*. Boca Raton, FL: CRC Press, pp. 201–205.

Gonzalez D (1990). Snake bites in domestic animals. *Toxicon* **28**, 149.

Kangstrom LE (1989). Snakebite in the dog and cat. *Svensk Veterinartidning* **41**, 38 (in Swedish).

Mayer S (1991). Poison: adder bite. *In Practice* **13(3)**, 126.

Yew / *Taxus baccata* and related plant species

The plant

Taxus baccata is commonly known as yew. The plant belongs to the Taxaceae family.

It is a slow-growing, evergreen shrub/tree which may grow to a height of about 20 m. It has a reddish-brown fibrous bark, and there may be more than one trunk to each tree. The leaves are needles up to 3 cm in length with two pale green bands on the underside. Dependent on the species they may range from golden yellow to dark green in colour. The male and female flowers grow on separate plants and it is only the female variety that will bear fruit. The flowers are so small as to almost be inconspicuous and appear on the plants from February to April.

The seed is about 5–7 mm long, brownish/purple in colour when ripe, green when unripe and ovoid in shape. It is enclosed in a fleshy aril that is green when unripe and red, or sometimes yellow, when ripe. The aril, which is often mis-identified as a 'berry' is usually about 7–11 mm long and about 7–8 mm wide and the seed is usually visible through it. The fruits are cup-shaped and contain sticky, mucilaginous flesh, that is reportedly sweet-tasting. They ripen from August to October.

Yew is commonly found on chalky/limestone soils in south and central England. It is native also to Wales. It is, however, found throughout the UK and is a common feature of many churchyards. It is also found in mainland Europe, particularly in areas of low altitude.

There are other varieties of the plant. The two most commonly encountered are:

(a) Irish yew (*Taxus baccata fastigiata*). This is a more erect and compact plant than the English yew. It has common use as a hedging plant.

(b) Japanese yew (*Taxus cuspidata*). This is an evergreen ornamental plant, with dark green glossy needle shaped leaves.

Occurrence of poisoning incidences

Since the launch of the VPIS in 1992, the London centre has received approximately 10 enquiries a year about yew. Twenty-three enquiries were received in 1997. Over 60% of these concerned suspected ingestion by dogs, the rest usually involving cattle. In the canine cases most remained asymptomatic, although some suffered profuse vomiting and salivation. All the dogs recovered.

Toxicity

All parts of the *Taxus baccata* plant are toxic, including dried clippings, with the exception of the fleshy red (or yellow) arils. It is thought that the other varieties mentioned above have similar toxicity to *Taxus baccata*.

According to the literature:

- 30 g of leaves is potentially fatal in a dog.
- 8 g plant material per kg body weight is quoted as a lethal dose in dogs.

Mechanism of toxicity

The toxic principle of the plant is its content of the alkaloids taxine A and B, which are found in all parts of the plant except the fleshy aril. Taxine B is cardiotoxic, with its effects due to inhibition of sodium and calcium currents. There is also an irritant volatile oil contained throughout the plant, as well as ephedrine and a cardiac glycoside named taxiphyllin. The gastrointestinal clinical effects are probably due to the irritant nature of the oils. The taxine alkaloids are non-irritant.

Kinetics and metabolism

Taxine alkaloids are rapidly absorbed from the gastrointestinal tract. They are metabolised in the liver and excreted as benzoic acid/conjugated hippuric acid.

Clinical effects

Clinical effects usually commence within 2 hours, although they may be delayed for up to 6 hours. The common effects in dogs are vomiting, diarrhoea, and excessive salivation, which all may be profuse. In some cases, the animals may have dilated pupils, lethargy, trembling, and ataxia.

In severe cases, hypothermia, bradycardia, hypotension, respiratory depression, convulsions and coma should be anticipated. Fatalities would usually result from heart or respiratory failure. In a canine case involving Japanese yew the animal became pyrexic, tachycardic, tachypnoeic and had dilated unresponsive pupils.

Taxine given to dogs produced ECG changes from wide QRS complexes to ventricular tachycardia and fibrillation.

Post-mortem findings

There is generalised inflammation of the stomach and presence of plant material. In cattle the findings have been an empty right heart, and the left heart, liver, spleen and lungs filled with dark, tarry blood.

Treatment

If only the fleshy aril has been ingested then no treatment is required. If any other part of the plant has been consumed and the animal has been presented within 3 hours then use of emetics followed by absorbents should be considered.

Emetics:

(a) Apomorphine	Dose:	0.05 mg/kg body weight i.v. or i.m.; 0.1 mg/kg body weight s.c.
(b) Xylazine	Dose:	0.2 mg/kg body weight i.v.; 0.5–1 mg/kg body weight i.m. or s.c.
(c) Ipecacuanha	Dose:	1–2 ml/kg body weight (maximum 20 ml) orally
(d) Soda crystal.		

Adsorbents:

(a) Activated charcoal	Dose:	2g/kg body weight orally
(b) BCK granules®	Dose:	6–18 g orally 2–3 times daily

Management thereafter is largely symptomatic and supportive. Particular care should be taken to ensure the animal is well hydrated. An observation period of 4–6 hours is recommended.

Diazepam may be given if there is any convulsant activity (dose: 0.5 mg/kg body weight i.v. repeated every 10 minutes up to three times if needed).

In serious cases where cardiac effects are present the administration of atropine may be of benefit.

Atropine dose: 30–100 μg/kg body weight s.c. or i.m.; 20 μg/kg body weight i.v.

Investigative

There are no clinically useful toxicological tests.

References and further reading

VPIS (London) past cases up to 97/58208.

Baker I (1992). Yew. *In Practice*, **14(1)**, 32.

Evans KL and Cook JR (1991). Japanese yew poisoning in a dog. *Journal of the American Animal Hospital Association* **27**, 300–302.

Hare WR (1998). Yew (*Taxus* spp.) poisoning in domestic animals. *Toxic Plants and Other Natural Toxicants*. Wallingford: CAB International, pp. 78–80.

General bibliography and references

Aiello SE (ed.) (1998). *The Merck Vetinary Manual* (eighth edition). Whitehouse Station: Merck and Co.

Allen DG, Pringle JK and Smith DA (1998). *Handbook of Veterinary Drugs*. Philadelphia, PA: Lippincott-Raven.

Andrews AH and Humphreys DJ (1992). *Poisoning in Veterinary Practice*. Enfield: National Office of Animal Health.

Bishop YM (ed.) (1996). *The Veterinary Formulary* (third edition). London: Pharmaceutical Press.

Bishop YM (ed.) (1998). *The Veterinary Formulary* (fourth edition). London: Pharmaceutical Press.

Blood DC and Studdert VP (1988). *Baillière's Comprehensive Veterinary Dictionary*. London: Baillière Tindall.

British Crop Protection Council (1997). *The Pesticide Manual* (11th edition). Farnham: British Crop Protection Council.

Cooper MR and Johnson AW (1998). *Poisonous Plants and Fungi in Britain Animal and Human Poisoning*. London: The Stationery Office.

Fraser CM, Bergerson JA, Mays A and Aeillo SE (eds) (1991). *The Merck Veterinary Manual* (seventh edition). Rathway: Merck and Co.

Frohne D and Pfänder HJ (1983). *A Colour Atlas of Poisonous Plants*. London: Wolfe Science.

Gfeller RW and Messonnier SP (1998). *Handbook of Small Animal Toxicology and Poisonings*. St Louis: Mosby.

Hayes WJ and Laws ER (eds) (1991). *Handbook of Pesticide Toxicology*. San Diego: Academic Press.

Henderson A (ed.) (1997). *The Henston Small Animal Veterinary Vade Mecum* (16th edition). Peterborough: Veterinary Business Development Ltd.

Humphreys DJ (1988). *Veterinary Toxicology* (third edition). London: Baillière Tindall.

Lorgue G, Lechenet J and Riviere A (1996). MJ Chapman (ed.), *Clinical Veterinary Toxicology* (English edition). Oxford: Blackwell Science.

Mabberley DJ (1987). *The Plant-Book*. Cambridge: Cambridge University Press.

National Office of Animal Health (1998). *Compendium of Data Sheets for Veterinary Products 1998/1999*. Enfield: National Office of Animal Health.

Osweiler GD (1996). *Toxicology*. Philadelphia: Lippincott, Williams and Wilkins.

Osweiler GD, Carson TL, Buck, WB and Van Gelder GA (1985). *Clinical and Diagnostic Veterinary Toxicology* (third edition). Dubuque: Kendall Hunt.

Postgraduate Committee in Veterinary Science, Sydney (1987). *Veterinary Clinical Toxicology* Sydney: Postgraduate Committee in Veterinary Science.

Royal Pharmaceutical Society (1996). *Martindale The Extra Pharmacopoeia* (31st edition). London: Royal Pharmaceutical Society.

Royal Pharmaceutical Society (1999). *Martindale: The Complete Drug Reference* (32nd edition). London: Pharmaceutical Press.

Tennant B (1994). *Small Animal Formulary*. Cheltenham: British Small Animal Veterinary Association.

Appendix I: Recommended holding for drugs used in management of poisoning cases

Unfortunately it seems to have become the norm to state the obvious in medical textbooks. So, with apologies, the editors would like to emphasise that this book is intended for veterinary clinicians, not for beginners, let alone amateurs. It does not give a discourse on the pharmacology of every treatment suggested, but relies on the reader's knowledge, experience and ability to consult the appropriate literature and texts.

The book, while very much UK based in the range of cases and possible toxicants discussed, takes a more global view of possible treatments. Whilst some British proprietary products (e.g. BCK® granules) are specifically mentioned, there has been no concerted attempt to fit the pharmacology within the potential 'pharmacy'. Thus, some of the products listed here are licensed for veterinary use, some are not. Different jurisdictions have different rules about 'off-label' use and about the use of unlicensed medicines. As this section is written the situation in the EU is drawing to a head and unless there is some dramatic change then – to take one example – the use of a fluorescein eye 'strip' to check for corneal ulceration in cattle (and probably horses) will have become a criminal offence by the time this book is published. The EU's 'Cascade Directive' is somewhat kinder to companion animals, but what drug can be used or should be used in each individual case must remain a matter of clinical judgement unique to that practitioner and that case. Whatever, we hope that access to the following, will assist once that judgement has been made.

Emetics
- Apomorphine
- Xylazine
- Syrup of Ipecacuanha
- Soda crystals – commercial 'washing soda' (that is sodium carbonate – *not* to be confused with caustic soda (sodium hydroxide), baking soda (sodium bicarbonate), etc.)

Adsorbents
- Activated charcoal
- BCK® granules

Anti-emetics
- Metoclopramide
- Acepromazine

Sedatives/anaesthetics

- Acepromazine
- Benzodiazepines (e.g. diazepam)
- Barbiturates (e.g. pentobarbitone)

Antidotal drugs

Zagreb® antivenom	(Adder bites)
Acetylcysteine	(Paracetamol)
Methionine	(Paracetamol)
Ascorbic acid	(Paracetamol)
Methylene blue	(Paracetamol/Nitrates/Chlorates*)
Cimetidine	(Non-steroidal anti-inflammatory drugs)
Sucralfate	(Non-steroidal anti-inflammatory drugs)
Ranitidine	(Non-steroidal anti-inflammatory drugs)
Famotidine	(Non-steroidal anti-inflammatory drugs)
Misoprostol	(Non-steroidal anti-inflammatory drugs)
Calcitonin	(Vitamin D, Calciferol)
Clodronate	(Vitamin D, Calciferol)
Desferrioxamine	(Iron)
Naloxone	(Opioids)
Atropine	(Organophosphates, Carbamates)
Beta-blockers	(Salbutamol, Theobromine)
Ethanol (20% solution)	(Ethylene glycol, Methanol, antifreeze)
Penicillamine	(Lead* and heavy metals*)
Sodium calcium edetate	(Lead* and heavy metals*)
Vitamin K_1	(Anticoagulants)

*Management for these agents is not discussed in this book.

Appendix 2: Case reporting

Below is a version of the case enquiry questionnaire used by the VPIS centres. We would be grateful to receive notification of any cases of interest handled by veterinarians. All data provided will be held in strict confidence.

Please complete a copy of this form and post to:

A Campbell
Veterinary Poisons Information Service – London
Medical Toxicology Unit
Avonley Road
London SE14 5ER, UK

If posting within the UK the Freepost service can be used. The address is:

Veterinary Poisons Information Service – London
FREEPOST
Medical Toxicology Unit
Avonley Road
London SE14 5BR

POISONING INCIDENTS INVOLVING ANIMALS

Date of Enquiry :   Time of Enquiry :

Case reference number :

1. DETAILS OF ANIMAL

a) Type:

b) Breed:

c) Animal name:

d) Age:

e) Weight:

f) Sex:

Male		Female		Pregnant	
Male (N)		Female (N)		Lactating	

g) Environment:

Domestic		Farm		Zoo/Collection	

h) Owners name / address :

i) Your case reference / name and address :

2. DETAILS OF AGENT

a) Name of agent / manufacturer :

Generic / Approved name	
Trade name	
Manufacturer name	
Manufacturer address	

b) Route(s) of exposure :

c) Quantity involved :

© VPIS

3. DETAILS OF INCIDENT

Where and how did the incident occur ?

4. CLINICAL EFFECTS AND TREATMENTS

a) Time from incident to onset of clinical effects :

b) Clinical effects observed and their period of duration :

c) Treatments instituted :

d) Laboratory investigations and results:

e) Outcome of case (if known) :

5. OTHER INFORMATION

Were any information services contacted to assist with management of this case ?

If 'yes' please state which :

© VPIS

Appendix 3: Normal values for cats and dogs

General
Cats

Heart rate (young)	130–240 beats per minute
Heart rate (adult)	100–240 beats per minute
Rectal temperature	101.5 ± 1°F/38.6 ± 0.5°C
Resting respiratory rate	26 breaths per minute (range 20–60)
Urine volume	10–20 ml/kg body weight/day

Dogs

Heart rate (young)	100–120 beats per minute
Heart rate (adult)	70–120 beats per minute
Rectal temperature	102 ± 1°F/38.9 ± 0.5°C
Resting respiratory rate (young)	20–22 breaths per minute
Resting respiratory rate (adult)	14–16 breaths per minute
Urine volume	20–100 ml/kg body weight/day

Biochemical and haemotological values
Cats

Base excess	+2 to −5 mEq/L	
Bicarbonate	15–24 mEq/L	15–24 mmol/L
Calcium	9.2–11.9 mg/dl	2.1–2.6 mmol/L
Chloride	117–123 mEq/L	117–123 mmol/L
Creatinine	1.2–2.1 mg/dl	106–186 μmol/L
Glucose	55–114 mg/dl	3.1–6.3 mmol/L
Haemoglobin	80–150 g/L	
Iron	68–215 μg/dl	12–39 μmol/L
pH (serum)	7.32–7.44	
pH (urine)	5.5–7.5	
Phosphorus	4.6–7.1 mg/dl	1.49–2.29 mmol/L
Potassium	4.0–4.5 mEq/L	4.0–4.5 mmol/L
Prothrombin time	7–12 s	
PTT (Partial thromboplastin time)	12–22 s	
Sodium	147–156 mEq/L	147–156 mmol/L

Dogs

Base excess	+6 to 0 mEq/L	
Bicarbonate	17–24 mEq/L	17–24 mmol/L
Calcium	8.7–11.8 mg/dl	2.18–2.95 mmol/L

Chloride	99–110 mEq/L	99–110 mmol/L
Creatinine	0.7–1.6 mg/dl	62–141 μmol/L
Glucose	55–102 mg/dl	3.1–5.7 mmol/L
Haemoglobin	120–180 g/L	
Iron	94–122 μg/dl	17–22 μmol/L
pH (serum)	7.31–7.53	
pH (urine)	5.5–7.5	
Phosphorus	2.8–7.7 mg/dl	0.9–2.45 mmol/L
Potassium	3.7–5.6 mEq/L	3.7–5.6 mmol/L
Prothrombin time	7–12 s	
PTT (Partial thromboplastin time)	12–15 s	
Sodium	137–149 mEq/L	137–149 mmol/L

Electrocardiographic data
Cats

P wave width	0.04 s
P-R interval	0.05–0.09 s
QRS width	0.04 s
QT interval	0.12–0.18 s

Dogs

P wave width	0.04 s
P-R interval	0.06–0.13 s
QRS width	0.05–0.06 s
QT interval	0.15–0.25 s

Other data
Cats

Gestation period	mean 63 days (range 58–70 days)
Suckling period	3–6 weeks

Dogs

Gestation period	mean 63 days (range 58–71 days)
Suckling period	3–6 weeks

Index

Lightning Source UK Ltd.
Milton Keynes UK
UKOW032341200613

212556UK00007B/201/P